Critical Perspectives in Happiness Research

Luka Zevnik

Critical Perspectives in Happiness Research

The Birth of Modern Happiness

Springer

Luka Zevnik
University of Ljubljana
Ljubljana
Slovenia

ISBN 978-3-319-04402-6 ISBN 978-3-319-04403-3 (eBook)
DOI 10.1007/978-3-319-04403-3
Springer Cham Heidelberg New York Dordrecht London

Library of Congress Control Number: 2014933270

Printed on acid-free paper

Springer is part of Springer Science+Business Media (www.springer.com)

I dedicate this book to my late father,
Ivo Zevnik.

Introduction: Towards a Critical Perspective in Happiness Research

Ever since Socrates (in Plato's Republic 352a) put forth his famous question about 'how we ought to live our lives,' happiness has not only represented one of the cardinal themes in Western thought, but it has also been perceived as being 'central to the point of human experience' (Nettle 2008, ix). While the intensity of interest in happiness in Western culture has varied across time, it is safe to argue that the second half of the 20th century and the beginning of the 21st are characterized by increased attention to this important but elusive theme. The list of self-help books offering various recipes for achieving happiness seems endless: *Happiness now!* (Holden 1999), *The Happiness Makeover: How to Teach Yourself to Be Happy and Enjoy Every Day* (Ryan 2005) and *Happy for no reason: 7 steps to being happy from the inside out* (Shimoff 2009), to name only a few.

The discourses about happiness have not only flooded the field of so-called pop-psychology, but also popular culture. Hollywood movies like the *Pursuit of Happiness* and *Eat Pray Love* testify that the cultural industries no longer sell only dreams, but also certain cultural representations of happiness. Journalists are also igniting the happiness bonfire: happiness and well-being have become common themes in both the electronic and more traditional print media like magazines and newspapers. The famous *Time* magazine, for example, dedicated a whole issue to happiness in 2005. Consumer culture is no exception, as we are increasingly sold not just products, but pure happiness. For example, Coca Cola's global campaign launched in 2009 was called *Open Happiness*, and the editorial in the IKEA 2010 catalog, entitled *Happiness*, promises 'a happier life at home' (provided that it is furnished with IKEA's furniture, of course).

On the other hand, people who doubt that happiness is a thing that can simply be bought and consumed have started engaging in various spiritual and healing practices more or less connected to new religious groups and movements that are increasingly penetrating the dominant culture. One can also educate oneself at an increasing number of conferences and seminars about happiness. From there, it is only a small step to therapy and so-called positive psychology, which opposes the traditional psychological focus on negative and pathological mental states and instead emphasizes the cultivation of positive ones.

A strong interest in happiness is also present in other academic disciplines. It is possible to observe a revival of interest in the philosophical tradition of the 'art-of-living,' which aims to provide philosophical answers to the question of how to lead a good and happy life. Meanwhile, more and more economists and politicians are acknowledging that the development of countries should not only be based on economic indicators like GDP, but it should also include indicators that show the well-being and happiness of their citizens. Last but not least, in the last few decades, a specialized interdisciplinary field called Happiness Studies, dedicated exclusively to the study and empirical research of happiness, has gained a lot of ground in academia.

All these recent developments, which constitute what Ahmed (2007/2008) calls 'the happiness turn,' represent the first reason why happiness figures as a topic worthy of an in-depth study. The second major reason to embark on a study of happiness is that evethough in the last decades we have witnessed an inflation of happiness research, there have been a very few attempts to provide a more critical perspective on happiness. In addition, the existent critical approaches within the so-called critical tradition/theory mostly focus on themes that are widely regarded as inherently problematic such as the problem of material inequalities, exploitation, racism and violence. While these are certainly important areas of critical analysis, I believe that, in addition to them, certain themes that are widely accepted as positive such as happiness can indeed be problematic and hence demand critical attention. In other words, even the themes (or one could even say precisely the themes) constituting our experience that are widely accepted as positive and unproblematic can (all the more easily) be connected to relations of power in society or better yet, can be employed in order to exercise certain forms of power. The next logical step from questioning the widely assumed "intrinsically positive nature of happiness" in Western culture is to also question its universality. Is happiness really a timeless universal experience?

The book offers an interdisciplinary exploration of the origins of happiness in the Western culture that questions these widespread assumptions. As such it provides a novel critical perspective on happiness that represents an alternative to the existent body of research dominated for the last 30 years mostly by psychology. In contrast to the prevalent quantitative empirical approach I intentionally do not start by articulating a construct/definition of happiness or well-being. Drawing from anthropology, cultural studies, critical sociology and cultural history I rather trace the unfolding of wider social processes and practices in the context of which happiness (along with its main characteristics) is defined (and made meaningful) by individuals, groups of individuals and institutions. It could hence be argued that the definition of happiness actually spans across the whole book and is not limited to a condensed "a priori definition". In this sense, the book is—epistemologically speaking—a call to "*return to happiness*". This paradigm shift aims to affirm wider historical, social and everyday meanings and practices related to happiness as vital focus of research. The call to "return to happiness" also implies that various scientific constructs and definitions of (subjective) well-being conceived in the ivory towers of academia should be stripped of their scientific myth about representing (more) objective models of happiness and must rather be recognized for what they are: merely one array of cultural constructions that have emerged as part of the current historical regime of happiness in Western culture.

In the first part of the book I offer a condensed overview of happiness research (Chap. 1) and an in-depth, critical review of the existent theories and research of happiness and its relation to culture (Chap. 2). To that end, the existent theories and empirical research concerning the connection between culture and happiness are critically examined and supplemented by insights from anthropology, cultural psychology, cultural studies, history and neuroscience. This provides the basis for the provocative argument that happiness is not universal but instead a culturally and historically specific experience that emerged in the 17th and the 18th century and that is characteristic only to the Western world. With the help of a novel interdisciplinary methodological framework developed in the end of the first part (Chap. 3), the second part of the book, expands upon this argument through an analysis of the social, religious, ethical and political processes that lead to the emergence of the experience of happiness.

The second part of the book is essentially the world's first Foucauldian inspired cultural history of happiness or put in Foucauldian terms: a genealogy of happiness. Genealogy of happiness is conducted with the help of the concept of experience used by the late Foucault to make sense of his entire opus. Following from this, genealogical analysis is conducted in every chapter in the second part along the three interconnected axes of experience that, according to Foucault, constitute the experience of any object: the axis of truth, the axis of relationship to the self and the axis of power. Accordingly, every chapter in the second part is organized into three main subsections, each corresponding to one respective axis of experience.

The second part of the book starts by examining how Christianity established salvation as the cardinal ideal of human existence and why such an ideal wasn't achievable in the present life (Chap. 4). The analysis of the medieval Christian experience is concluded by arguing that it cannot be simply equated with the experience of happiness, which only emerged in the 17th and 18th century, when the ideal of human existence increasingly started to be pursued in the present life.

The first steps towards the birth of happiness are traced back to the times of the Renaissance and the Reformation movement (Chap. 5), which were still, however, mainly characterized by the Christian experience. In addition to the existent and still prevalent Christian ideal of salvation, the Renaissance movement (starting in the 15th and 16th centuries) and the Reformation movement (starting in the 16th century) introduced what I call the problematization of (good) feeling and the affirmation of everyday life, which later resulted in the experience of happiness. The problematization of (good) feeling on earth and the affirmation of everyday life for some time, therefore, coexisted with the preceding and still dominant idea of salvation, until in the 17th century the former started to slowly but surely dominate the latter.

In Chap. 6 I argue that it was precisely this transformation (in which good feeling on earth in connection with the affirmation of everyday life started becoming the primary ideal of human existence) that represented the first major development, which marked the birth of the modern experience of happiness. The second such major development was that the ideal of human existence not only became possible already in this world, but also that it became perceived as entirely achievable with human efforts. Since the birth of happiness also established the basic structure for all later forms of happiness in Western culture, the illumination of this process is relevant not only because it can support the argument of the historical and cultural character of happiness, but also because it represents a valuable point of departure for any further inquiries into manifestations of happiness in our culture. In this regard Chap. 7 briefly outlines the development from the birth of happiness to its contemporary manifestations. Here it has to be noted that the books' main focus is on the birth of happiness in the 17th and the 18th century. Consequently the analysis of the developments after the birth of happiness condected in Chap. 7 is less in-depth and should be seen as a point of departure of future research. As an example of the latter I conduct an analysis of modern consumer culture that is depicted as one of the main strategies of happiness in contemporary western societies. In the Conclusion (8) I recapitulate the main steps leading to the birth of happiness and argue that happiness has represented one of the central themes guiding the processes of modernization that have fundamentally determined what we experience today. Following from this, (the birth of) happiness is presented as essential to our understanding of a broader context in which important aspects of individual and social life—such as consumer culture, the modern state, economic system, science and technology, idea of progress, etc.—have emerged in the West.

Ljubljana, 2013

Acknowledgements

I am grateful to my family for their love and continuous support. I thank Leja and her open heart for being there for me and with me during long hours of writing.

I thank Chris Barker and Peter Stanković for their guidance and trust in me. Also, I couldn't have done it without all of my colleagues and friends who gave me inspiration of various kinds. I am especially grateful to Blaž Vrečko Ilc for his sincere friendship and our extensive Foucauldian debates.

Last but not least, I would like to thank Esther Otten and Hendrikje Tuerlings at Springer for their warm and professional approach to making this book a reality.

Contents

Part II The Birth of Happiness

Part I
The Return to Happiness

Chapter 1
Overview of Happiness Research

This chapter will provide a condensed overview of the major approaches for the study and research of happiness that have started multiplying especially after the 1970' and try to illuminate their main characteristics. Since the cardinal aim of this chapter is not to provide an inclusive intellectual history of the idea of happiness in the western culture, we shall not explore the works of specific authors in-depth. Rather, the aim is to map out a theoretical and research field within which it will be possible to situate all the major approaches for the study and research of happiness in the western culture. Within this field we are then going to position our own theoretical point of departure for the study of happiness that will be predominantly focused on the connection between culture, happiness and relations of power.

Happiness and Philosophy

The philosophical approach initiated by Socrates's question about how we ought to live our lives has had the longest and the richest tradition of studying happiness in the western culture out of which all other "non-philosophical" approaches have later evolved. Within the modern classification of philosophy happiness is positioned in the domain of moral philosophy. According to the editors of a recent philosophical reader on happiness, the theme of happiness actually represents 'a central topic of moral philosophy' (Cahn and Vitrano 2008, p. vii). In this sense, argue Cahn and Vitrano (2008, p. vii), the entire history of ethics could even 'be viewed as a set of variations on the theme of happiness'.

The philosophical approach to happiness deals with the nature, source and value of happiness and it includes questions like: What is happiness? What are its causes and conditions? How to determine the criteria for what counts as causes, conditions and source of happiness? How to live a good and happy life? Is something like ultimate happiness even possible? Is happiness necessary for a worthwhile life? Is it sufficient? Does happiness depend on one's state of mind, one's consequences or both? Etc.

L. Zevnik, *Critical Perspectives in Happiness Research*,
DOI 10.1007/978-3-319-04403-3_1, © Springer International Publishing Switzerland 2014

Ever since the Antiquity it is hard to find a single philosopher in the history of western thought who wouldn't tackle at least one of the above questions. While in more general discussions about happiness within (moral) philosophy all of these questions are usually closely connected, it is nevertheless possible to identify two specific sub-approaches that vary according to the emphasis given on particular lines of questioning. Insofar as the majority of explicit philosophical takes on happiness pertain to one of these sub-approaches they deserve a closer inspection.

The oldest approach which elaborates on the Socrates' question how we ought to live our lives is usually referred to as the tradition of philosophy as a way of life. Due to its practical appeal it is often also called the tradition of art-of-living (Nehamas 1998, p. 2), which according to Dohmen (2003, p. 351) forms a part of the subfield of moral philosophy called normative ethics. Art of living 'is a form of self-direction with a view to the good life' (Dohmen 2003, p. 351) that stresses the connection between logos and bios, between theory and practice. Namely, argues Nehamas (1998, p. 2), within the philosophy of art-of-living 'what one believes and how one lives have a direct bearing on one another'. According to Nussbaum (1994), Hadot (1995) and Nehamas (1998) the art-of-living philosophy has predominated above all other forms of philosophy in the ancient Greek and Roman times. Antique philosophers like Socrates, Plato, Aristotle, Epicurus, Seneca etc. have all provided and pursued different visions on how to live a happy life.

With the rise of Christianity in the second half of the first millennia, art-of-living philosophy has mostly given way to Christian theology. In the contemplations of theologians like St. Augustine, John Cassian, Gregory of Nyssa and St. Aquinas the classical art-of-living (or the care of the self as Foucault (2000a, p. 288) calls it) has mostly been transformed and integrated into Christian renouncement and deciphering of the (earthly) self. In this sense happiness as the ultimate ideal of human existence was replaced by the notion of bliss (beatitude) that belonged to the realm beyond this world.

Within modern philosophy the tradition art-of-living regained some of its original momentum in the works of philosophers like Michel de Montaigne, Blaise Pascal, Artur Schopenhauer, Søren Kierkegaard, Friederich Nietzsche, Pierre Hadot, Michele Foucault etc. We have to note, however, that according to several prominent modern philosophers such as Kant (in Nehamas 1998, p. xii), Nietzsche (1997) and Nehamas (1998), art-of-living tradition has never reacquired the predominant role it had occupied in Antiquity and represents only a marginal current in modern philosophy.

Already Kant (in Nehamas 1998, p. xii) in the The Philosophical Encyclopaedia was aware that modern philosophy seldom fails in following the art-of-living imperative for harmonizing theory and practice towards a good and happy life: 'When will you begin to live virtuously, Plato asked an old man who was telling him that he was attending a series of lectures on virtue. One must not just speculate forever; one must one day also think about actual practice. But today we think that those who live as they teach are dreamers'. Nietzsche (1997, p. 187) was even more harsh in his critique of the practical sterility of the modern institutionalized philosophy: 'The only critique of a philosophy that is possible and that proves something, namely trying to see whether one can live in accordance with it, has never been taught at universities: all that has ever been taught is a critique of words by means of other words'. Nehamas (1998) observes that the situation diagnosed by Kant, Nietzsche and later also Foucault (2005) persists in contemporary philosophy. Still, he argues, philosophy has only 'few practical implications for everyday life' (Nehamas 1998, p. 1). In order to at least partly re-activate the art-of-living tradition in contemporary philosophy Nehamas' (1998, p. 2) book 'aims at opening a space for a way of doing philosophy that constitutes an alternative, though not necessarily a competitor, to the manner in which philosophy is generally practiced in our time'. For Nehamas (1998, p. 2) this implies recognizing that a conception of philosophy as a way of life 'exists, study how it survives in some major modern philosophers, and see that it is what some of us are still doing today'. And indeed according to several authors involved in the art-of-living themselves (see Cottingham 1998; Dohmen 2003; Kekes 1995, 2002), art-of-living is gradually gaining ground in contemporary moral philosophy. This "revival of art-of-living philosophy" is part of a larger trend of increased interest in the theme of happiness towards the end of the twentieth and the beginning of the twenty-first century in the western societies, which Ahmed (2007/2008) calls 'the happiness turn'.

While the tradition of art-of-living is predominantly concerned with ways of achieving individual happiness, there is another notable sub-approach of philosophy of happiness that emerged much later than the art-of-living and that extended the philosophical discussion of the quest for happiness to the realm of the collective. In Antiquity it was held that happiness was only achievable by way of a prolonged and intensive cultivation of one's life that was reserved for the rarified ethical elite. Following from this, philosophy concerned with happiness was predominantly equated with art-of-living understood as an individual exercise aimed at achieving individual happiness in the present life. With the introduction of the notion of original sin Christianity universally refused the possibility of attaining the ideal of human existence on earth replacing the art-of-living philosophy with theology and Christian asceticism. The break with the centuries long tradition of sin and the decisive step towards the philosophy of collective happiness was only made in the seventeenth century by a rationalist current in the Christian tradition. The so-called Deism and natural theology transposed the universalizing message of Christianity from 'universal sinfulness' to the idea of a 'universal providential order created by the merciful God for the mutual benefit and happiness of all of its inhabitants both in heaven and on earth. On such bases it was possible for the first time in the history of western culture to conceive of a philosophy of communal or public happiness most lucidly captured in the famous maxim 'the greatest happiness for the greatest number'. The philosophy of communal happiness culminated in the enlightenment utilitarian philosophy, which directly connected happiness with the maximization of earthly sensual pleasure.

The main innovation of utilitarian philosophy for the study of communal happiness was the idea that 'if maximizing happiness is the point of individual lives, then the point of systems of government and economy should be to maximize collective or aggregate happiness' (Nettle 2008, p. ix). Dedicated to the enlightenment vision of human and social progress and their belief that human affairs can be examined with a set of objective numerical and mathematical gauges initially developed for the study of natural laws, utilitarian philosophers have formulated various algorithms to measure (the progress towards) individual and collective happiness. In spite of the fact that they lacked precise data for their algorithms, the philosophy of communal happiness laid the foundations for what has later become a science of happiness.

The Science of Happiness

For millennia, argues Ed Diener (2008, p. 245) the father of empirical happiness research, the study of happiness 'was the domain only of philosophers, religious scholars, and armchair thinkers'. On the crossroads of psychology and sociology a new approach to happiness has emerged in the western culture in the 1960', which claims that in comparison to the speculative nature of inquiry in philosophy, it can provide systematic, empirical and scientific accounts of happiness. At least indirectly marked by philosophical approach to happiness, similarly also the science of happiness has two main sub-approaches: one that mainly focuses on individual happiness and one that focuses on (measuring and providing) collective happiness.

Considering its main emphasis on individual happiness[1] the so-called positive psychology pioneered by psychologist Martin Selingman (2003) could be seen as a scientific version of art-of-living philosophy. Contrary to the approach of traditional psychology that is dedicated to the 'amelioration of psychopathology' (Ryan and Deci 2001, p. 142), positive psychology focuses on the scientific study of happiness, well-being and positive emotions. Positive psychologists clearly acknowledge that they 'have not invented the study of happiness, well-being, or strengths' (Positive Psychology Center 2010). In their view the most important contribution of their approach to the study of happiness has rather been

> to make the explicit argument that what makes life most worth living deserves its own empirically based field of study, to provide an umbrella term that brings together isolated lines of theory and research, to promote the cross-fertilization of ideas in related fields through conferences, summer institutes and research grants, to develop a comprehensive conceptual view of broad notions of happiness, to bring this field to the attention of various foundations and funding agencies, to help raise money for research, and to firmly ground assertions on the scientific method (Positive Psychology Center 2010).

In this sense 'positive psychology is the scientific study of the strengths and virtues that enable individuals and communities to thrive' (Positive Psychology Center 2010). According to the Positive Psychology Center (2010) such 'objective,

[1] Even though positive psychology is undoubtedly also concerned with some aspects of communal happiness and emphasizes a good social context as one of important conditions for individual happiness, it is primarily concerned with individual happiness.

empirical research' of happiness can 'help people make more informed choices' that are supposed to lead them to a happier life.

If positive psychology could be regarded as a scientific version of philosophy of art-of-living, empirical research of happiness could be perceived as the practical actualization of the utilitarian philosophers' dream to objectively measure (collective) happiness[2]. And indeed Veenhoven (1997), one of the pioneers of empirical happiness research does recognize the utilitarian legacy of empirical happiness research both in terms of its dedication to social progress towards the greatest happiness for the greatest number as well as in terms of the ideal of scientific objectivity in measuring it.

Empirical researchers of happiness emphasize that for as long as happiness has been 'a playground for philosophical speculation', the understanding of happiness has 'remained speculative and uncertain' (Veenhoven 1997, p. 1). In their view it was only the development of quantitative scientific methods such as survey-research that enabled happiness to be approached in objective scientific way. That, however, was only the condition for the rise of empirical happiness research. The most important reason for its rise was the increasing awareness emerging in the 1960' 'that, just as positive affect is not the opposite of negative affect well-being is not the absence of mental illness' (Cacioppo and Berntson 1999 in Ryan and Deci 2001, p. 142) that in the last decades resulted in a rapid and vast development of the interdisciplinary field now known as happiness studies[3].

According to Ryan and Deci (2001, p. 146) empirical happiness research has derived from two different perspectives on happiness and well-being that 'have led to quite different types of inquiry concerning the causes, consequences, and dynamics of well-being': 'the hedonic approach, which focuses on happiness and defines well-being in terms of pleasure attainment and pain avoidance; and the eudaimonic approach, which focuses on meaning and self-realization and defines well-being in terms of the degree to which a person is fully functioning' (Ryan and Deci 2001, p. 141). While the debate between hedonic and eudaimonic theorists has been intensive ever since Antiquity and is far from coming to a final resolution, most of researchers working on the empirical field would agree that strictly speaking happiness is not a concept entirely appropriate for the scientific approach. Following from this happiness is usually either equated or replaced with the term well-being. Authors working from the hedonic perspective like Diener (2008, p. 692) see the scientific construct of well-being as a more technical term for happiness, which in their view 'allows for a certain degree of precision in measuring the fuzzier, folk concept of happiness'. While as a consequence they do not refuse the concept of happiness as such (after all they still speak of happiness studies), eudaimonic

[2] Although positive psychology is also grounded in the scientific research and measurement of happiness we have decided to treat the two approaches separately on account on different emphasis they put on individual and collective happiness.

[3] Insofar as the positive psychology approach is grounded in empirical research and measurement of happiness the two approaches in many respects overlap. In this sense positive psychology can be also regarded as a part of happiness studies.

researchers on the other hand usually avoid the concept of happiness as being insufficient for capturing their (normative) vision of human well-being.

These differing understandings of happiness and well-being adopted by various empirical happiness researchers 'have led to quite different types of inquiry concerning the causes, consequences, and dynamics of well-being' (Ryan and Deci 2001, p. 146). Let us first look at the so-called hedonic perspective, on which the earliest and the most prevalent approach to empirical happiness research has been founded.

For researchers who work from the hedonic perspective happiness 'concerns the experience of pleasure versus displeasure broadly construed to include all judgments about the good/bad elements of life' (Ryan and Deci 2001, p. 144). In other words they are interested in 'what makes experiences and life pleasant and unpleasant' (Kahneman et al. 1999, p. ix). 'Although there are many ways to evaluate the pleasure/pain continuum in human experience', observe Ryan and Deci (2001, p. 144), the predominant research method of the hedonic approach has been the assessment of the so-called subjective well-being or SWB. Subjective well-being 'consists of three components: life satisfaction, the presence of positive mood, and the absence of negative mood, together often summarized as happiness' (Ryan and Deci 2001, p. 144).

Within SWB research happiness is thus 'conceived as overall life-satisfaction and measured using self-reports' (Veenhoven 2006, p. 1). In his review articles Diener (1984), Diener et al. (1997) identifies three cardinal characteristics in the study of SWB. The first is that 'the field covers the entire range of well-being from agony to ecstasy' (Diener et al. 1997, p. 1). The second one is that 'SWB is defined in terms of the internal experience of the respondent' (Diener et al. 1997, p. 1). SWB research therefore doesn't impose an 'external frame of reference' when assessing SWB but rather gives 'the ultimate authority' to the respondent (Diener et al. 1997, p. 1). In other words 'the assumption behind self-reports of SWB is that the respondent is in a privileged position to report his or her experience of well-being' (Diener et al. 1997, p. 2). And the third characteristic is that 'the field focuses on longer-term states, not just momentary moods'. That is, 'SWB research is interested in relatively enduring feelings of well-being, not just fleeting emotions' (Diener et al. 1997, p. 1).

The most common method for assessing SWB 'is through self-report surveys in which the respondent judges and reports his life satisfaction, the frequency of her pleasant affect, or the frequency of his unpleasant emotions' (Diener et al. 1997, p. 2). Below is an example one such questionnaire developed by Pavot and Diener (1993) called Satisfaction With Life Scale (SWLS):

Using the 1–7 scale below, indicate your agreement with each item by placing the appropriate number on the line preceding that item. Please be open and honest in your responding.

7—Strongly agree

6—Agree

5—Slightly agree
4—Neither agree nor disagree
3—Slightly disagree
2—Disagree
1—Strongly disagree
In most ways my life is close to my ideal.
The conditions of my life are excellent.
I am satisfied with my life.
So far I have gotten the important things I want in life
If I could live my life over, I would change almost nothing.

Due to the potential shortcomings of self-report measures (like response biases, memory biases, and defensiveness), some researchers are trying to develop other ways of measuring SWB. According to Diener (1997, p. 3) alternative methods for measuring SWB include: the research of 'people's frequency of smiling, their ability to recall positive versus negative events from their lives, and reports from the target respondent's family and friends'. In addition to standard questionnaires, there are also 'alternative methods based on self-reports such as interviews and the experience sampling method (mood reports are collected at random moments over a period of weeks)' (Diener 1997, p. 3).

There are also attempts to measure happiness by cognitive science. Neuroscientists like Richard Davidson (Davidson et al. 2004) use brain imaging to observe the cerebral activity of happy people and try to identify brain areas associated with happiness. In addition, biological psychologist John Cacioppo (Cacioppo et al. 2008) uses electrodes to measure tiny movements in facial muscles associated with various emotions. He then shows pleasant, neutral and unpleasant pictures to his participants and observes the differences between the reactions of people reporting different levels of happiness. Yet another biological method for assessing happiness is through measuring human biochemistry—hormones circulating in the blood and in the brain.

In spite of all the new innovative attempts to research happiness, observes Diener (2008, p. 252), self-reports still remain 'the most frequent way we measure well-being'. In Diener's (2008, p. 252), view other methodologies of SWB research can only 'complement self-reports in their strengths' enabling what Eid and Larsen (2008, p. 5) call 'multimethod assessment' of SWB: 'Although each of the non-self-report methods has its own shortcomings, psychologists can gain an especially strong assessment of SWB by using several methods in tandem because in this way a number of response artifacts can be eliminated' (Diener et al. 1997, p. 3). However, even multimethod assessment of SWB, acknowledges Diener (2008, p. 253), can only provide 'a reasonably accurate measure of happiness' that is still far from being 'perfect'.

According to Veenhoven (1997) SWB research can and is used for several purposes. The first and the most elementary use of SWB research is 'to estimate apparent quality of life in a population' where a high level of happiness in a population 'suggests that the quality-of-life is good' (Veenhoven 1997, p. 2). This is typically done, further explains Veenhoven (1997, p. 2) 'to assess whether there is a social problem that requires policy intervention'. The next application of SWB research is 'monitoring social progress and decline over time' and 'to assess policy effects; in particular for evaluating attempts to improve quality-of-life' (Veenhoven 1997, p. 3). In this sense the effects of policy interventions 'can be measured by changes in happiness before and after, or by differences in happiness between beneficiaries and non-beneficiaries' (Veenhoven 1997, p. 3). And last but not least, argues Veenhoven (1997, p. 3), 'the most interesting use of empirical happiness research is the validation of ideas about conditions for the good life, and related ideas about the good society'.

Contrary to the hedonic standpoint on happiness, a eudaimonic perspective 'refers to well-being as distinct from happiness per se' (Ryan and Deci 2001, p. 145). Based on Aristotelian philosophy, 'eudaimonic theories maintain that not all desires—not all outcomes that a person might value—would yield well-being when achieved. Even though they are pleasure producing, some outcomes are not good for people and would not promote wellness' (Ryan and Deci 2001, p. 146). For authors within the eudaimonic perspective subjective happiness cannot therefore simply be equated with well-being. Rather they understand human well-being in Aristotelian terms of human flourishing. Namely, either as 'the striving for perfection that represents the realization of one's true potential' (Ryff 1995, p. 100), as living in accordance with one's true authentic and expressive self (Waterman 1993), or as living 'with the requirements of human nature' (Fromm 1981, p. xxvi, 2007).

Based on their critique of hedonic visions of well-being, researchers working from the eudaimonic perspective challenge 'SWB models of well-being as being of limited scope where positive functioning is concerned, and specifically that SWB is often a fallible indicator of healthy living' (Ryan and Deci 2001, p. 146). Instead some of them have developed their own measures of well-being based on the eudaimonic perspective often reffered to as Eudaimonic Well-Being (EWB). Ryff (1989) for example proposes the measure of Psychological Well-being (PWS), Ryan and Deci (2000) support their Self-determination theory (SDT) research and Waterman et al. (2010) use the Questionnaire of Eudaimonic Well-being (QEWB). While initially these methods represented somewhat less prominent current in empirical happiness (well-being) research dominated by hedonic approach and SWB meassurements, the eudaimonic perspective is rapidly gaining ground. Considering that the EWB is seen by its proponents not only as a complement but also as a contrast to the more established SWB, in the recent years we are witnessing a lively development of EWB methods and a vibrant theoretical discussion between the two different approaches to the study of the quality of life (see for example Kashdan et al. 2008; Waterman et al. 2010).

The Economy of Happiness

On the bases of certain insights of empirical happiness research some economists have opened a new field of research within economy called the economy of happiness or 'happiness economics' that 'is gaining increasing attention among economists, psychologists, sociologists and the public' (Bruni and Porta 2007, p. xvi). In particular economy of happiness was inspired by the so-called happiness paradox[4] introduced by Easterlin (1974) who is consequently considered to be the father of economy of happiness. Easterlin (1974), used the data of extensive, quantitative, longitudinal, human happiness research to argue that when a particular individual or society reaches a certain level of economic wealth, any further increase in income does little or nothing to increase the level of happiness and well-being. The main focus of economics of happiness then is 'explaining the happiness paradoxes' that 'calls into question some of the basic tenets of contemporary economics' like considering well-being as a simple function of income or seeing the increase of GDP as the main vision for the development of societies (Bruni and Porta 2007, p. xvii). Based on their specific explanations of the happiness paradox economists working in the "happiness tradition" propose different new policies and encourage governments to govern and allocate resources in accordance with what they believe to be the reasons behind the paradox.

Above we have described the main approaches for the study of happiness that have evolved in the western culture. The book will primarily focus on the tradition of empirical happiness research, which—as we have argued—approaches happiness not as an ethical theme like philosophy but sees happiness as an object of scientific research. Within this empirical tradition we will give special emphasis to the connection between happiness and culture. There are two major reasons for such a particular focus. The first is connected with the fact that the empirical approach hasn't yet been systematically critically reflected and the second is that treating happiness as the object of research provides a point of departure for questioning the widespread assumption of intrinsically unproblematic nature of happiness in the Western culture.

[4] After its author the happiness paradox is sometimes also called the Esterlins's paradox.

Chapter 2
Happiness, Culture and Relations of Power

The crux of this chapter will be to explore the relationship between happiness, well-being and culture. To that end, we shall examine the existent theories and empirical research about the connection between culture and happiness and try to identify the moments at which they could be criticized and complemented. Our central aim will be to question happiness and well-being as universal experiences and to suggest that they are culturally and historically specific/singular notions and experiences, the constitution of which is also closely connected to the workings of power.

Cross-National Measurements of Happiness and Culture

In spite of the fact that the complexity and magnitude of the empirical study of happiness has grown at a steady pace since the 1960s, it was only towards the end of the twentieth century that the field of happiness studies became increasingly interested in the relation between culture and happiness. Initial reflections on happiness in the context of culture have been predominately catalyzed by the methodological issues in cross-national empirical research on subjective well-being. Comparisons of reported levels of SWB between various national states could undoubtedly be regarded as one of the central issues in empirical research on happiness from its beginning in the 1960s up until now (Veenhoven 1997). Cantril's cross-national study on 'Pattern of Human Concerns,' for example, already included happiness as a variable in 1965 (see Cantril 1965). Cantril's research, and the majority of the numerous other comparative research studies of SWB that followed, addressed various methodological issues related to comparing happiness across countries such as sampling and the problems of measurement. It was not until the beginning of the 1980s that the influence of culture came to be seen as one of the possible methodological issues. Namely, Ostroot et al. (1981) analyzed the quality-of-life perceptions held by the inhabitants of two culturally different cities: Springfield Illinois, USA and Aix-en-Provence, France. The research of Ostroot et al. was certainly not the first to observe significant differences in levels of SWB across nations, but it was one of the first that clearly identified a methodological issue that later become designated as

L. Zevnik, *Critical Perspectives in Happiness Research*,
DOI 10.1007/978-3-319-04403-3_2, © Springer International Publishing Switzerland 2014

the 'cultural bias' (Veenhoven 1991). The cultural bias implies that the comparative differences in the appreciation of life do not necessarily pertain to the actual differences between levels of happiness, but are rather a result of cultural variations that influence peoples' perceptions of their well-being. Ostroot et al. (1981), and later Baumeister (1991), argued, for example, that a higher level of happiness reported by Americans could be connected to the fact that their culture places happiness much higher up on the list of values than the French. In other words, their cultural context encourages Americans to present themselves as happier than they actually are. Another methodological reservation posed by later research was that the survey-based measurement of happiness could be distorted in cultures that are less familiar with the concept or that have a significantly different concept of well-being (see Ouweneel and Veenhoven 1991, p. 2; Mathews and Izquierdo 2009, p. 8).

Growing discussions around the influence of culture on the measurement of SWB gradually turned cross-national comparisons of SWB into cross-cultural comparisons. A notable step in that direction has been the *Culture and Subjective Well-being* reader edited by Diener and Suh (2000). The main focus of the reader is the identification of differences in SWB between cultures/states. To that end, the authors examine cultural factors that influence SWB (e.g. Triandis 2000; Oishi 2000) and 'ask whether specific societal conditions generally lead to SWB in the nations of the world' (Diener and Oishi 2000). The authors also place much emphasis on methodological issues regarding different modes of survey-based cross-cultural comparisons of happiness, which include 'the question of measurement,' 'issue of causality,' problems with 'defining and measuring the cultural and societal variables that predict well-being,' 'sampling,' etc. (Diener and Suh 2000, pp. 5–8).

It is not unusual for researchers to employ different methods for the measurement of SWB across cultures[1]. What is of far greater importance for our discussion is that authors working in happiness studies differ significantly in their perception of the degree of influence of culture on happiness. While in general (especially after the publication of *Culture and Subjective Well-being* reader) most of the authors in happiness studies acknowledge a certain connection between culture and happiness, they are certainly not univocal in their understanding about the nature and the extent of that relation (Diener 2007, pp. 693–695). Or, as Ryan and Deci (2001, p. 161) have put it: 'researchers within the field of well-being are grappling with an issue that cross-cuts all social sciences, namely that concerning cultural relativism versus universals in human nature'.

Universal Notions of Well-Being and Culture

While there are two extreme positions on the connection between culture and happiness (one that sees happiness and well-being as universal—independent from culture—and the other that sees happiness as entirely culturally specific), the majority

[1] For more on different methods of measuring SWB across cultures, see Diener and Suh (2000, pp. 5–8) and Diener (2007).

of empirical researchers opt for the middle path, maintaining that some components of well-being are universal and the others, culturally specific (Diener 2007, pp. 693–695). In this sense, most of them would agree with Diener and Suh's (2000, p. 4) editorial in *Culture and Subjective Well-being*, which only perceives culture as one of the factors influencing SWB: 'SWB reflects to some degree how much people are living in accord with evolutionary imperatives and human needs, but also represents judgments based on the particular norms and values of each culture'.

We agree with Tiberius (2004), who argues that regardless of how they perceive the relation between culture and happiness, those researchers who are relying on survey-based cross-cultural comparisons of (subjective) well-being are assuming a universal notion of well-being on which they can ground their research. While Tiberius (2004, p. 293) and, according to her, 'most philosophers,' working in the area of well-being actually try to articulate and support such universal notions of well-being, we, on the other hand, will suggest that the ambition of philosophers and other theoreticians and researchers of well-being to 'clear the ground for a universal notion of well-being' (Tiberius 2004, p. 293) should not be accepted without scrutiny.

According to Tiberius (2004, p. 293), a formal philosophical project in the area of well-being that aims to formulate universal notions of well-being is not 'undermined by the kinds of cultural differences that have been discovered and that, therefore, there might be a universal notion of well-being'. Tiberius (2004) builds her principal argument solely on the basis of empirical cross-cultural SWB comparisons, which only 'discover differences in the causes, source, or perhaps even the components of well-being' (Tiberius 2004, p. 295). She argues that in order for such comparisons 'to proclaim that these are differences about well-being, they must presuppose an account of the nature of well-being that is the referent of a concept we share with other cultures' (Tiberius 2004, p. 295). As a consequence, Tiberius believes (2004, p. 295), cultural differences in the sources or causes of well-being do not undercut universal notions of well-being that are 'attempting to provide the criterion for what counts as a source or cause'. On the contrary, according to Tiberius (2004), SWB researchers need to assume such a universal notion and, consequently, 'defending such an account is one of the main projects of philosophers' working on the formal analysis of well-being.

We certainly agree with Tiberius that empirical survey-based cross-cultural comparisons of SWB do need to presuppose a universal notion of well-being. Moreover, we believe that Tiberius's argument is even more far-reaching, proving that actually any attempt to compare happiness or well-being across different cultures means that the researcher is knowingly or unknowingly assuming a universal notion of well-being. Without such an assumption, Tiberius rightly argues (2004, p. 295), 'Differences between goods pursued by various cultures could not be reported as differences that have to do with well-being'.

Yet, in our view, this is not enough to ultimately maintain a universal notion of well-being nor of happiness, with which well-being is usually equated within empirical happiness research. Namely, we shall argue that Tiberius's defense of universal notions of well-being is plausible only for as long as culture is perceived solely as influencing the causes and source of well-being. To that end, let us first take a closer look at the most recent insight into the connection between culture and well-being from the so-called cultural perspective in happiness studies, on the basis of which we are going to build our argument on.

The Cultural Perspective in Happiness Studies

Authors with a background in cultural psychology that constitutes the so-called cultural perspective in happiness studies (like Kitayama and Markus 2000; Lu and Gilmour 2004; Uchida et. al. 2004; Pflug 2008) argue that the influence of culture reaches beyond the sources or causes of well-being. Rather, they comprehend culture in the broadest sense as 'a particular way of life' (Williams 1983, p. 90) and, consequently, do not only consider culture as one of the factors in the understanding of well-being and happiness, but rather as the cardinal factor: 'culture can be a major force constructing the conception of happiness and consequently shaping its subjective experiences. In particular, members of different cultures may hold diverse views of happiness, covering definitions, nature, meaning and ways to strive for SWB' (Lu and Gilmour 2004, p. 271). Of course, this does not mean ignoring factors like 'evolutionary imperatives and human needs' and 'human nature' (Diener and Suh 2000, p. 4, 5). Instead, even factors like evolutionary imperatives, human needs and human nature that might seem "natural" and "universal" are manifested in culturally specific ways:

> Just as people cannot live in a general way and must of necessity live in some set of culture-specific ways, a person cannot just be well in a general way. The very nature of what it means to be well or to experience well-being takes culture-specific forms. What it means to feel good or to live a good life requires being able to realize culturally mandated ways of being (Kitayama and Markus 2000, p. 114, 115).

According to Kitayama and Markus (2000), and later also Lu and Gilmour (2004), the two compounds of SWB—"the subject/self" and "well-being"—that constitute any experience of happiness are not general, universal or ahistorical phenomena and experiences, but rather historically and culturally specific social constructions that are established through 'cultural practices and meanings' (Kitayama and Markus 2000): 'The cultural perspective assumes that psychological processes—in this case, the nature and experiences of SWB—are thoroughly culturally constituted. Thus, culture and SWB are most productively analyzed together as a dynamic of mutual constitution' (Lu and Gilmour 2004, p. 271). What, therefore, counts as well-being 'depends on how the concepts of "well" and "being" are defined and practiced' in a particular culture or a society (Kitayama and Markus 2000, p. 115). This means that 'members of different cultures may hold diverse views of well-being, covering definitions, nature, meaning and ways to strive for SWB' (Lu and Gilmour 2004, p. 271), where specific conceptions of happiness form specific experiences of happiness. Moreover, 'culture also influences SWB in the way it gives shape and form to the self' (Lu and Gilmour 2004, p. 272). Here, we have to note that the cultural construction of the self 'is socially mediated, meaning that it occurs in conjunction with the construction of social relationships' (Kitayama and Markus 2000, p. 114).

Besides the influence of culture on both the subject/self and the conceptions of happiness, there is also a mutual connection between the self/subject and SWB, meaning that 'the self stands at the junction of subjective well-being and culture. Culture provides 'form and shape to the self' and specific definitions of both 'well and being,' which in mutual influences produce how individuals feel and think about various aspects of their lives—the central research issue of SWB' (Suh 2000, p. 63). 'To the extent that the relevant social world is arranged and practiced differently, incorporating different cultural models of what is good, what is moral, or what is self,' Kitayama and Markus conclude (2001), 'well-being may assume forms other than those currently described and documented in the psychological literature'.

Claiming that well-being and happiness are culturally and historically specific phenomena does not imply that cultures are closed self-sufficient units independent from each other. On the contrary, cultures that directly or indirectly interact with each other always influence each other. The idea of so-called inter-cultural diffusion also holds in the case of happiness and well-being. Lu and Gilmour's (2004, p. 272) qualitative comparative research in Euro-American and Asian culture, for example, has clearly identified 'cultural fusion' in the field of well-being:

> In a time of cultural fusion, people living in the collectivist East are learning to adopt cultural values, self-views, beliefs, attitudes and behaviors from the West. Consequently, they may now subscribe to both individual and socially oriented conceptions of SWB, and have access to both Eastern and Western repertoires of striving for SWB. A parallel trend in the individualist West in the opposite direction may be less salient due to a certain asymmetry in cross-cultural impact, not least because the very nature of core values at issue inclines Westerners to impact more aggressively on their environment, including other cultures.

Here, it is important to add that according to the cultural perspective, the cultural construction of happiness is not only culturally specific, but also historically specific, for both the self/subject and cultural conceptions of happiness are 'grounded in historically nurtured ideologies and religious ideas' (Uchida et al. 2004, p. 227). As a consequence, an analysis of the cultural constitution of experience of happiness has to also include 'the history of the culture' (Kitayama and Markus 2000, p. 114) in which it is grounded. Such a historical analysis was demonstrated by Lu and Gilmour (2004), who argued that Asian conceptions of SWB are largely marked by 'Confucian, Taoist, and Buddhist' historical influences, whereas the Euro-American conceptions are marked by their Christian legacy.

Ethnocentrism and Universal Notions of Well-Being

Taking the cultural perspective into account, it is possible to claim that Tiberius's arguments for a universal notion of well-being are plausible for only as long as the analysis of the relation between culture and well-being remains limited to empirical survey-based cross-cultural comparisons that indeed are only capable of discovering cultural differences in causes and sources of well-being. Insofar as empirical cross-cultural research on well-being fails to identify and explain the nature of well-being, Tiberius believes that it has to be established by philosophers who formulate it as a universal notion of well-being. However, Tiberius (2004, p. 301) also rightly acknowledged that 'more dramatic differences' identified by cross-cultural research in well-being 'would be evidence that the two words we thought referred to the same concept (of well-being L.Z.), in fact refer to two different things'. As we have seen above, a cultural perspective that combines qualitative empirical evidence with theoretical analysis has revealed that the differences between cultures indeed are 'more dramatic' than discovered by quantitative SWB research and acknowledged by Tiberius (2004): 'It is not that different things make people happy in different cultural contexts—that is obviously the case. More significantly, it is the ways of "being well" and the experience of well-being that are different' (Kitayama and Markus 2000, p. 115). That is, 'the very nature of what it means to be well or to experience well-being takes culture-specific forms' (Kitayama and Markus 2000, p. 114). Insofar as there are not only the causes and sources of well-being that differ across cultures but also its nature[2], by articulating universal notions and definitions of well-being, philosophers, researchers or theoreticians of happiness are in fact superimposing their own particular conception of nature of well-being based on meanings and practices of their cultural background on other cultures. In other words, by advocating or trying to articulate universal notions and definitions of well-being, they are inescapably caught in a form ethnocentrism, which corresponds to a 'process by which values and ways of seeing the world that are founded in one culture are used to comprehend and judge another' (Barker 2004, p. 63).

Since quantitative survey measurements and comparisons of well-being need to presuppose such universal concepts and definitions of happiness, they are also susceptible to the charge of ethnocentrism. By placing 'contemporary understandings of psychological and subjective well-being' in a 'cultural and historical context,' Christopher (1999, p. 141) has put forward several convincing arguments to support 'the hypothesis that, despite intentions to be value-neutral, subjective well-being is actually normative; its very design presupposes values and assumptions that are central to Western culture' (Christopher 1999, p. 146). Even though Christopher mostly refers to the psychological SWB research, which was prevalent at the time of the writing of his article, we believe that his arguments are equally valid for all perspectives in empirical happiness research that advocate or assume universal notions of well-being[3]. According to Christopher (1999, p. 141), empirical survey happiness research (and, in our view, other theoretical and research perspectives in happiness studies also) problematically presupposes 'ontological and liberal individualism as notions of the self and as normative prescriptions for the good or ideal person'. Ahmed (2007/2008, p. 10) is close to Christopher's position, arguing that

[2] Empirical evidence for this argument can be found both in the work done within the cultural perspective in happiness studies (see for example Kitayama and Markus 2000; Lu and Gilmour 2004; Uchida et al. 2004; Pflug 2008; Oishi et al. 2013) and in the research of anthropology of well-being (see Mathews and Izquierdo 2009).

[3] This includes the eudemonic approach to empirical happiness research (EWB) that examines well-being based on the "universalized" Aristotelian vision of well-being, which is clearly tied to the Western cultural context.

'the science of happiness relies on a *very* specific model of subjectivity, where one knows how one feels, and where the distinction between good and bad feeling is secure, forming the basis of subjective as well as social well-being'. And so are Kitayama and Markus (2000, p. 153): 'often as innocuous and well-intended as they are, various attempts to apply theories of happiness that are implicitly grounded in Western ideas of progress, liberalism, egalitarianism, and freedom to other cultural contexts may not reveal, but distort, lived experiences of the people in those cultures'.

Rather than uncritically relying on biased universal notions of well-being, Christopher argues (1999, p. 149), therapists, theoreticians and researchers of happiness ought to be conscious of the fact that 'understandings of psychological well-being necessarily rely upon moral visions that are culturally embedded and frequently culture-specific'. As a consequence, 'the idea of developing entirely culture-free measures, theories or interventions is seriously misguided' (Christopher 1999, p. 149). If we (as researchers and theoreticians of happiness and well-being) 'believe that we are discovering universal and ahistorical psychological truths rather than re-interpreting and extending our society's or community's moral visions,' Christopher further warns (1999, p. 149), 'then we run the risk of casting non-Western people, ethnic minorities, and women as inherently less psychologically healthy'.

The 'anthropology of well-being,' conceived with the publication of the first anthropological reader on happiness, and edited by Mathews and Izquierdo (2009, p. 8), is also 'highly skeptical' towards quantitative survey-based research of happiness, 'seeing them as inevitably ethnocentric in their use of Western-derived survey instruments to compare a range of societies across the world'. In spite of the fact that these survey-based studies are becoming more sophisticated, anthropologists insist that universal notions and scales used by quantitative researchers 'privilege some cultural conceptions over others' (Mathews and Izquierdo 2009, p. 8). As a consequence, they believe that 'American or Western conceptions of well-being are insufficient to understand well-being in a range of societies across the globe, and are thus insufficient as a basis for the cross-cultural comparison of well-being' (Mathews and Izquieredo 2009, p. 9). Similar to the cultural perspective in happiness studies, anthropology adopts a cultural constructionist approach[4]: 'happiness, as we have argued, is subjective and culture-bound, and cannot easily be ascertained by any universal measures. Different societies may adhere to different culturally and linguistically constructed concepts of happiness, making cross-societal comparison more or less problematic' (Mathews and Izquierdo 2009, p. 5).

Anthropologists of well-being see the answer to the problem of ethnocentrism inherent in philosophical universal notions of well-being and empirical survey research in cultural relativism that has been one of the most important tenets of their discipline since the start of the twentieth century. Before we can explore what cultural relativism brings to the research of happiness, we first have to clarify the 'problem with an unswerving cultural relativism' in relation to well-being as raised

[4] This similarity is quite obvious considering the fact that cultural psychology was actually born out of a strand of twentieth-century anthropology (see LeVine 2007).

by Diener and Suh (2000, p. 5). While 'respecting many differences between countries,' Diener and Suh (2000, p. 5) and Diener (2007) are reluctant about what they call an 'all-out cultural relativism' because according to them, it is 'too accepting of terrible people and sick societies'. With the help of anthropology, we have to observe that Diener and Suh (2000) have apparently based their position on cultural relativism on an erroneous understanding of the concept. Claiming that the problem with cultural relativism is 'that every outcome is as good as every other; a Hitler is judged to be as good as Francis of Assisi' (Diener and Suh 2000, p. 5) points to an obvious confusion between the concepts of cultural relativism and moral relativism. According to Marcus and Fisher (1986, p. 32), such misuses of the concept emerge from the fact that cultural relativism 'has all too often been portrayed as a doctrine rather than as a method and reflection on the process of interpretation itself'. While an extreme position of moral relativism, conceived as rejecting universal moral truths, could indeed lead to Diener and Suh's radical claim on cultural relativism, for anthropologists the concept instead corresponds to a methodology that follows the guidelines that there is

> no one best or most rational way to organize society; that different cultures had evolved different constellations of values and social mechanisms; that it is often more realistic to try to learn alternative ways of organizing societies by observing other cultures than by ivory-tower speculation about reforming society; that cultural values cannot be ethically judged in abstract philosophical terms, but must be evaluated in terms of their actual effects on social life (Marcus and Fischer 1986, p. 170).

Anthropologists, hence, persistently defend against 'critics who charge that relativism asserts the equal validity of all value systems, thus making moral judgments impossible, and that in its insistence on fundamental respect for cultural differences among human societies, it has paralyzed all schemes of generalization, by which the progress of any science must proceed' (Marcus and Fischer 1986, p. 32).

Criticism of Survey Happiness Research

According to the anthropologists of well-being, the cross-cultural comparison of survey data is not only ethnocentric, but also 'leaves out too much to be fully credible' (Mathews and Izquierdo 2009, p. 6). According to (Mathews and Izquierdo 2009, p. 6) this is because 'surveys do not ask respondents to talk about their senses of well-being in their own words'. Rather, further argue (Mathews and Izquierdo 2009, p. 6) 'they ask for informants' closed-ended answers to fixed questions, as translated into different languages. This not only ignores how individuals express their own senses of their lives, but also ignores how different languages and cultures conceive of well-being in different ways[5]'. In other words, surveys 'reify what can be measured and ignore what cannot be measured' (Mathews and Izquierdo 2009,

[5] This is also confirmed by Wierzbicka's (2004) cross-linguistic and cross-cultural research on happiness.

p. 8). According to anthropologists of well-being, the only way to adhere to the methodological premises of cultural relativism and to avoid the inherent incompleteness of survey research is to conduct ethnographic research in the cultures of interest, 'which can provide the social and cultural context without which well-being in a given society cannot be fully understood' (Mathews and Izquierdo 2009, p. 250):

> Anthropologists specialize in understanding, through extended fieldwork, the complex cultural meanings that exist within a given society. They may be especially well situated to understand a given society's particular language formulations of well-being and to reveal, through close ethnographic description, how these play out in people's daily lives, words, and worlds (Mathews and Izquierdo 2009, p. 9).

Following from this, Mathews and Izquierdo warn (2009, p. 6), we have to be extremely careful when comparing different cultures in terms of well-being: 'it is indeed possible to make a comparison of different societies as to well-being, as long as this is done in a careful, culturally sensitive way. This can be done through what we in this book term soft comparison, comparison based not on—or at least not solely on—bald statistics placed side by side, but rather on all the nuances of socio-cultural context ethnographically portrayed' (Mathews and Izquierdo 2009, p. 6). In this sense, anthropologists of well-being consider their approach as an 'empirical antidote to the straitjackets of comparison adhered to by some other disciplines, such as economics and psychology, which more or less insist on a common standard of measurement for all societies' (Mathews and Izquierdo 2009, p. 248).

Even though the cultural perspective in happiness studies does not proclaim to be following cultural relativism,[6] nor does it explicitly criticize survey methods on account of their ethnocentrism, it could be argued that it adheres to all the major methodological tenets of cultural relativism as understood by anthropologists of well-being:

> A cultural psychological approach does not automatically assume that all behavior can be explained by the same set of constructs and measures, and enquires first whether a given construct is meaningful and how it is used in a given cultural context. In other words, a Western conception of SWB should not be superimposed on other cultures; instead, indigenous conceptions of SWB bred in particular cultural contexts should be unraveled and systematically mapped out (Lu and Gilmour 2004, p. 271).

The cultural perspective also agrees with the anthropology of well-being that 'statistical measures of well-being are not inherently flawed, but they are inherently incomplete' (Mathews and Izquierdo 2009, p. 250):

> The literature on well-being has so far been based on large surveys. Although useful in revealing general descriptions, this methodology has inherent limitations. The cultural perspective presented here suggests that cultural meanings are often tacit—they are not recognized by the person who engages in them, and they therefore are unlikely to be revealed in any survey data. A variety of reasons underlie this problem of survey methodology. The

[6] Perhaps the reason behind this is connected with the fact that they are trying to avoid the charge of moral relativism that could be based on the misunderstanding of their position on cultural relativism.

> most important is that cultural meanings are embodied in patterns of cultural practices and conventions. Such practices and conventions are often tacit, normative, carrying little, if any, subjective significance. Yet, they are a significant contributor to subjective well-being. They provide the framework within which individuals, singly or collectively, seek to achieve cultural adaptation in order to attain a state of well-being. Research can benefit from dense descriptions of the lived world of the peoples under study, and then by bringing this cultural knowledge to bear on the theories and methods developed to test those theories (Kitayama and Markus 2000, p. 153).

While the anthropology of well-being is almost exclusively in favor of the ethnographic method, a cultural perspective is open to a variety of both quantitative as well as qualitative methods. To support their thesis and compare different cultural constructions of well-being, researchers from the cultural perspective use different quantitative (e.g. Kitayama and Markus 2001; Uchida et al. 2004) and qualitative research methods (e.g. Lu and Gilmour 2004; Pflug 2008). The latest research, however, seems to lean more towards the qualitative side, as it is more suitable for exploration of cultural meanings and practices that enter in the cultural construction of happiness. Lu and Gilmour (2004) and Pflug (2008), for example, have asked their research group to write essays on the theme 'What is happiness?' and, thus, tried to extrapolate the meanings respondents with a different cultural background attributed to happiness.

Happiness as Culturally and Historically Specific Experience

Above, we have discussed whether happiness and well-being can be considered as universal notions and experiences or if they are culturally specific. As shown, within the traditional empirical happiness research, the connection between culture and happiness has initially been explored as a purely methodological issue within cross-national comparative happiness measurements. Gradually, culture has become a relevant factor to be considered in order to explain and measure the differences in levels of happiness between nations and cultures. However, amongst happiness researchers and theoreticians, there are still notable differences in understanding the relationship between culture and happiness. Tiberius (2004) has showed that regardless of how they perceive the relation between culture and happiness, all researchers who are relying on survey-based cross-cultural comparisons of SWB are assuming a universal notion of well-being on which they can ground their research. While Tiberius (2004) and, according to her, most philosophers and researchers working in the area of well-being, try to support or assume universal notions of well-being, we, on the other hand, have questioned them. Namely, we have argued that Tiberius's defense of universal notions of well-being is only valid for as long as differences between cultures are perceived solely in terms of causes and sources of well-being. Since the cultural perspective in happiness studies and anthropology of well-being have discovered more fundamental differences between cultures, we have questioned universal notions of well-being and instead considered happiness and well-being as culturally and historically specific social constructions established through cultural meanings and practices. We have stressed that by articulating or assuming universal formal notions and definitions of well-being, philosophers, researchers or theoreticians of happiness are in fact superimposing their own culture-bound criteria for what counts as well-being onto other cultures. While on account of this, survey-based cross-cultural comparisons of (subjective) well-being are charged with Western ethnocentrism, especially by the anthropologists, both anthropology and the cultural perspective in happiness studies agree that statistical measures of well-being are inherently incomplete, leaving out too much to be fully credible. As a consequence, they both (explicitly or implicitly) try to follow the cultural constructionist thesis and methodological tenets of cultural relativism that imply that societies should be explored and evaluated on their own unique terms. Following from this, they are both more in favor of qualitative methods such as ethnography and unstructured interviews that, in their view, can provide a more accurate and verifiable scientific picture of happiness and well-being than the quantitative survey research.

Happiness and the Promise of Neuroscience

Available empirical data on the differences in the nature of well-being across cultures and the danger of ethnocentrism evident on the universalist side suggest a considerable amount of scepticism towards universal notions of happiness and well-being. Yet, it has to be noted that this important issue is still not entirely resolved. The promise of the rapidly developing field of neuroscience alone suggests that we have to allow the possibility of an empirical discovery of a more general underlying structure in the nature of well-being, which may be universal. In the future, the field of neuroscience, which has only started to develop an interest in happiness (see, for example, Berridge and Kringelbach 2010), seems to offer a promise of providing new empirical methods for measuring happiness that would not be plagued by the problems of survey methods identified above. Time will show how the development of neuroscience might contribute to the discussion about the possibility of a universal notion of well-being. Currently, the 'neuroscience of happiness is still in its infancy' facing difficult questions regarding the relation of the nature of well-being (and its components) to underlying brain systems (Berridge and Kringelbach 2010). For now, Berridge and Kringelbach explain, 'while some progress has been made in understanding brain hedonics' neuroscience has 'still not made substantial progress toward understanding the functional neuroanatomy of happiness' (2010, p. 673). Until neuroscience (or any other scientific discipline for that matter) provides firm empirical evidence of possible universal structures in the nature of happiness and well-being the cultural perspective therefore presents itself as a more reasonable alternative.

As a consequence we mostly approve of the theoretical insights and the methods for the research of happiness and well-being introduced by the anthropology of well-being and cultural perspective and believe that they have made important contributions to the discussion about the connection between culture and happiness. However, it needs to be noted we that their approaches have certain theoretical as well as empirical weaknesses and lacunae, which have to be addressed.

Problematic Issues with the Cultural Perspective in Happiness Studies and Anthropology of Well-Being

Providing valuable ethnographic analysis about well-being in different cultures, the anthropology of well-being is undoubtedly more "culturally sensitive" than the survey methods of cross-cultural happiness measurement, which it so vigorously criticizes on account of their ethnocentricity. Yet, in our view, and insofar as anthropologists of well-being also adhere to a universal notion of well-being, they are also susceptible to a subtle form of ethnocentrism. Namely, the anthropology of well-being articulates a universal notion of well-being in the form of a 'broad definition' of well-being (Mathews and Izquierdo 2009, p. 5):

> Well-being is an optimal state for an individual, community, society, and the world as a whole. It is conceived of, expressed, and experienced in different ways by different individuals and within the cultural contexts of different societies: different societies may have distinctly different culturally shaped visions of well-being. Nonetheless, well-being bears a degree of commonality due to our common humanity and interrelatedness over space and time. Well-being is experienced by individuals—its essential locus lies within individual subjectivity—but it may be considered and compared interpersonally and interculturally, since all individuals live within particular worlds of others, and all societies live in a common world at large.

Even though anthropologists of well-being try to formulate their definition on the basis of cultural relativism, they are still imposing certain universal criteria for what counts as well-being. Namely, associating a universal definition of well-being with the word 'optimal,' which derives from the Latin *optimus*, meaning best, can be ethnocentric, considering that research from the cultural perspective in happiness studies has indicated that 'the notion that it is good to increase the good and to decrease the bad may be cultural' and that 'it is rooted in the European-American ideology of linear progress' (Kitayama and Markus' 2001, p. 153).

With the help of insights from the cultural perspective, we have also argued in a similar way above that universal notions of well-being that formulate the criteria of what counts as a source or a cause of well-being articulated by philosophy (and assumed by survey research on well-being) are problematic on account of their ethnocentrism. However, even though the cultural perspective does not explicitly articulate universal notions or criteria of well-being, a thorough reflection reveals that insofar as it claims to be discovering and explaining differences in cultural constructions of happiness and (subjective) well-being, it too might be somewhat problematic. That is, in order to be able to discover differences in cultural constructions of happiness, a cultural perspective has to implicitly articulate a broader, universal notion of well-being that formulates criteria for what counts as a cultural construction of well-being on the ground of which it can claim to be observing the cultural construction of the same phenomena in different cultures. In other words, just as survey research needs to assume universal criteria for what counts as causes of well-being in order to discover differences in the causes and sources of well-being across cultures, a cultural perspective needs to articulate certain universal criteria for what counts as the cultural construction of well-being in order to be able to discover differences in the cultural construction of well-being across cultures.

In our view, universal notions of well-being implicitly or explicitly assumed by the cultural perspective and anthropology of well-being are more of a theoretical issue and far less problematic than the ethnocentrism and incompleteness of quantitative survey-based cross-cultural measurements of happiness. Nevertheless, this does not mean that it should not be addressed. We believe that universal notions in a cultural perspective in happiness studies and that the anthropology of well-being in fact persist as part of a larger issue, which is that both approaches fail to acknowledge all the consequences of the cultural construction thesis and apply them also to the(ir own) research on happiness and well-being. In addition, there are some other aspects of the study and research of happiness and well-being that are either problematic or not (adequately) covered by the cultural perspective and anthropology of well-being, which include issues like relations of power related to the cultural construction of happiness and the need for a more thorough historical analysis. While in our view these issues and lacunae do not undermine the bulk of their analytical and methodological contributions to the study and research of happiness, we believe that their approaches could nevertheless be significantly improved and complemented.

To that end, we shall draw from the so-called postmodern or interpretative anthropology to argue that the consequences of the cultural construction thesis (in happiness studies) are not only methodological, but also epistemological and ontological, and try to examine what this brings to the study and research of happiness and well-being. With the help of cultural studies, we shall then argue that the cultural construction of happiness is also connected to the relations of power in society, which hasn't yet been recognized by the existent approaches of empirical happiness research. Last but not least, we will emphasize the importance of historical analysis in the understanding of the construction of happiness and note that the mode in which it has been undertaken so far has ignored certain important aspects of the historical constitution of experience of happiness in Western culture.

The Consequences of the Cultural Construction (of Happiness) Thesis

Insofar as the cultural perspective and anthropology of well-being perceive the cultural construction thesis mostly on the methodological level, they are essentially implying that by explaining and understanding the process of the cultural construction of happiness and well-being that they are providing a more verifiable scientific picture of happiness and well-being than the quantitative survey research. Some anthropologists 'have doubted the possibility of ever achieving the rigor of a hard scientist, partly because they could not experiment with human beings,' and 'partly because of the immense complexity of human interaction'; nevertheless, a scientifically accurate description indeed 'was an ideal to which they usually aspired' (Barrett 1996, p. 150). While the anthropology of well-being and the cultural perspective in happiness studies as the (grand)daughter of anthropology still mostly seem to follow this ideal, the postmodern anthropology, on the other hand, has very much questioned the strict scientific foundations of anthropology and its ability to provide accurate descriptions of the world and of (other) cultures. For postmodern anthropologists like Clifford (1986), Marcus and Fischer (1986) and Tyler (1986), 'it was no longer the case of science being unobtainable due to technical obstacles' (Barrett 1996, p. 150). Rather, their position against the ideal of a science of culture was more theoretically profound as they challenged it on ontological, epistemological and ethical grounds.

Providing a theoretical framework for postmodern anthropology, Rabinow (1986) draws mostly from Rorty[7] (1979), who works his case against modern epistemology, portraying it as 'an accidental, but eventually sterile turning in Western culture' (Rabinow 1986, p. 234). Rorty (1979, p. 315) understands epistemology as a study of mental representations that is not universal, but rather a historically singular event in European philosophy after the seventeenth century, driven by a desire to find firm foundations of knowledge: 'the desire for a theory of knowledge is a desire for constraint—a desire to find "foundations" to which one might cling, frameworks beyond which one must not stray, objects which impose themselves, representations which cannot be gainsaid'. The modern notion of epistemology on which modern science is founded, thus, focuses on the problem of the relation between external reality and internal representations. According to Rorty (1979), Rabinow explains (1986, p. 235), such a relationship towards truth was established by Descartes whose 'conception of knowing rests on having correct representations in an internal space, the mind'. In this sense:

> to know is to represent accurately what is outside the mind; so to understand the possibility and nature of knowledge is to understand the way in which the mind is able to construct such representations. Philosophy's eternal concern is to be a general theory of representations, a theory which will divide culture up into the areas which represent reality well, those which represent it less well, and those which do not represent it at all (despite their pretense of doing so) (Rorty 1979, p. 3).

However, Rabinow explains (1986, p. 235), it was only by Kant, who 'established as a priori the Cartesian claim that we have certainty only about ideas,' that 'the eventual demarcation of philosophy from science was made possible by the notion

[7] Rorty (1979) is certainly not the only representative of what is often called the postmodernist critique of modern science. In the following chapter, we shall also examine Foucault's original criticism of modern science. Insofar as we will be dealing with the critique of modern science mostly in the context of anthropology and Foucauldian theory, we shall not focus on other notable examples of this approach such as Lyotard's (1984) famous critique of grand/meta narrative of modern science.

that philosophy's core was a "theory of knowledge," a theory distinct from the sciences because it was their foundation' (Rorty 1979, p. 132).

While epistemology primarily remains the foundation of modern science, there is an alternative tradition in modern thought that does not seek 'to improve epistemology but to play a different game' (Rabinow 1986, p. 236). Namely, Rorty (1979) follows authors like 'Wittgenstein, Heidegger and Dewey' who 'are in agreement that the notion of knowledge as an accurate representation, made possible by special mental processes, and intelligible through a general theory of representation, needs to be abandoned' (Rorty 1979, p. 6). In this sense, Rorty replaces epistemology and the quest for improving it for an approach based on the notions of anti-representationalism and anti-foundationalism:

> Anti-representationalism is understood to mean that the relationship between language and the rest of the material universe is one of causality, not of adequacy, of representation or of expression. That is, we can usefully try to explain how human organisms come to act or speak in particular ways, but we cannot beneficially see language as representing the world in ways, which more or less correspond to the material world. There are no chunks of language that line up with or correspond to chunks of reality. Above all, there is no Archimedean vantage-point from which one could verify the universal 'truth' of any correspondence between the world and language. The anti-foundationalism that follows from this argument suggests that we cannot ground or justify our actions and beliefs by means of any universal truths. We can describe this or that discourse, chunk of language, as being more or less useful and as having more or less desirable consequences. However, we cannot claim it to be true in the sense of correspondence to an independent object world. We can examine the way that the word 'truth' is used, what makes a particular truth claim acceptable to us and our routine deployment of 'mundane realism'. However, we cannot give an epistemological account of truth and must steer clear of philosophical claims about transcendental and metaphysical truth (Barker 2002, p. 10).

Yet, as Rabinow rightly observes (1986, p. 240), in his theory of anti-representationalism and anti-foundationalism, Rorty ignores the category of power, which determines which knowledge is—in spite of the fact that it ultimately lacks foundation in the objective reality—established as truth by a 'wide range of disparate, but interrelated, social and political practices that constitute the modern world'. In this sense, we agree with Rabinow (1986, p. 241) who—as a consequence—sees Foucault[8] as an important upgrade of Rorty's refusal of epistemology: 'many new possibilities for thought and action are opened up if we follow Rorty and abandon epistemology (or at least see it for what it has been: an important cultural movement in Western society) and follow Foucault in seeing power as productive and permeative of social relations and the production of truth in our current regime of power'. Anti-representationalism and anti-foundationalism, combined with the understanding of the relations of power connected to the production of knowledge, thus, imply skepticism towards any universal and objective knowledge about the world including the knowledge of modern science. Instead, we must accept the notion of positionality (or, in Nietzsche's words, perspectivism), which is used to indicate

[8] In the following, we shall also examine Foucault's own original refusal of modern epistemology that is not covered by Rabinow (1986).

> that knowledge and 'voice' are always located within the vectors of time, space and social power. Thus, the notion of positionality expresses epistemological concerns regarding the who, where, when and why of speaking, judgment and comprehension. That is, specific acculturated persons make truth-claims at an exact and distinct time and place with particular reasons in mind. Consequently, knowledge is not to be understood as a neutral or objective phenomenon, but as a social and cultural production since the 'position' from which knowledge is enunciated will shape the very character of that knowledge./…/ It follows from this argument that we cannot ground or justify our actions and beliefs by means of any universal truths. We can describe this or that discourse as being more or less useful and as having more or less desirable consequences. However, we cannot claim it to be true in the sense of correspondence with an independent object world (Barker 2004, p. 154).

The research strategy following from the notions of anti-representationalism, anti-foundationalism and positionality, Rabinow argues (1986, p. 241), is that 'we need to anthropologize the West; show how exotic its constitution of reality has been; emphasize those domains most taken for granted as universal (this includes epistemology and economics (and also happiness studies; LZ)); make them seem as historically peculiar as possible; show how their claims to truth are linked to social practices and have, hence, become effective forces in the social world'.

Applying this research strategy to the research of happiness and well-being means to question happiness and well-being as universal notions and phenomena in an even more radical sense than done by anthropology of well-being and the cultural perspective in happiness studies. It includes absolutely refusing all universal notions and definitions of well-being, even the ones that constitute the ground to discover differences in cultural constructions of happiness and well-being assumed by anthropology and the cultural perspective in happiness studies. Strictly speaking, this means that insofar as well-being and happiness are notions and experiences specific to Western culture (both in terms of everyday conceptions as well as in terms of conceptions articulated by researchers and theoreticians), we must analyze them precisely as that: singular cultural phenomena that emerged only within Western culture. In other words, when speaking of happiness and well-being either in terms of research or everyday experience, we have to acknowledge that we are speaking of particular concepts and experience that have only emerged in Western culture and that are specific only to Western culture. Literally, this is a call to "return to happiness" with which we want to imply affirming happiness as the primary and the most relevant focus of study and research. In this sense, various scientific constructs and definitions of (subjective) well-being conceived in the ivory towers of academia should be stripped of their scientific myth about representing (more) objective models of happiness and must rather be recognised for what they are: merely one array of cultural constructions that have emerged as part of a wider historical regime of happiness in Western culture.

Completely refusing universal notions of well-being, we also cannot research happiness and well-being in other cultures, as this would inescapably imply superimposing our own culture-bound criteria for what either counts as causes or sources of well-being or for what counts as a cultural construction of well-being onto other cultures. This does not suggest that we cannot conduct research in other cultures. What it does suggest, however, is that without assuming a universal notion of well-being, we can only carefully and sensitively research certain cultural constructions in other cultures for which we can conditionally claim that they constitute a similar thing to happiness and well-being, but certainly not the same thing[9]. What has to be assumed in this case, then, is not an a priori universal notion of well-being that articulates criteria for what counts as well-being, but an ontological position of cultural and social construction of reality. That is, to account for the differences across cultures in this sense, we do not need an analytical basis on which differences regarding a preconceived universal phenomenon (like well-being) can be discovered, but an analytical foundation that can explain how being is culturally and historically constituted as different kinds of experience.

Since there is 'no Archimedean vantage-point from which one could verify the universal "truth" of any correspondence between the world and language' (Barker 2002, p. 10), there is no such thing as objective knowledge about happiness and well-being even within Western culture. That is, we can only talk of happiness in terms of specific notions and experience socially constructed through meanings and practices in Western culture.

The foundations for such a methodological approach in anthropology were laid by Geertz (1973), the forefather of postmodern anthropology, who proposed the switch in the anthropological analysis from structure and causality to meaning and interpretation. In this sense, culture corresponds to a system of signs and symbols or 'an assembly of texts'[10] (Geertz 1973, p. 448). While the cultural perspective and anthropology of well-being also focus on cultural meanings and practices, they—as we have argued above—failed to acknowledge all the consequences of the interpretative approach and, thus, remain within the epistemological framework of modern science. Following from this, the cultural perspective and the anthropology of well-being see their methods as producing more accurate in-depth descriptions of well-being and happiness across cultures. In contrast, for an interpretative anthropology that is attuned to the notion of positionalism analysis is not an objective scientific description but an well informed interpretation. As such it is closer to a literary method of interpreting texts than an objective scientific method: 'anthropological writings are themselves interpretations, and second and third ones to boot. (By definition, only a "native" makes first-order ones: it's his culture.) They are, thus, fictions; fictions in the sense that they are "something made," "something fashioned"… not that they are false' (Geertz 1973, p. 15). Perceiving ethnographies as fictions, Clifford explains (1986, p. 6), does not mean that they are 'something merely opposed to truth,' but rather 'suggests the partiality of cultural and historical truths, the ways they are systematic and exclusive'. 'If "culture" is not an object to be described, nor is it a unified corpus of symbols and meanings that can be definitively interpreted' (Clifford 1986, p. 19), it follows that ethnographic truths trying to interpret other cultures as well as our own are 'constructed,' 'inherently

[9] For pragmatic purposes, the word could be translated, provided of course that this is done with the reflection of the position from which this translation is taken.

[10] Text here is perceived in the broadest sense as anything that conveys meaning and requires interpretation.

partial—committed and incomplete' (Clifford 1986, p. 6). That is, 'even the best ethnographic texts—serious, true fictions—are systems, or economies, of truth'[11] (Clifford 1986, p. 7).

Taking the notion of positionality into account, anthropology, thus, 'no longer speaks with automatic authority for others defined as unable to speak for themselves' and has to acknowledge that 'ethnographic work has indeed been enmeshed in a world of enduring and changing power inequalities, and it continues to be implicated' (Clifford 1986, p. 9).

The ideal of cultural relativism that claims to be evaluating cultures in their own unique terms is, thus, ultimately unattainable. When researching cultures, postmodern anthropologists argue, we can then only try to critically reflect on the position from which the research is conveyed: 'now ethnography encounters others in relation to itself, while seeing itself as other' (Clifford 1986, p. 23). Following from this, 'we do not need a theory of indigenous epistemologies or a new epistemology of the other. We should be attentive to our historical practice of projecting our cultural practices onto the other' (Rabinow 1986, p. 241). In this sense, Marcus and Fischer argue (1986, p. 32), 'interpretative anthropology might best be understood as the reinvigorated and sophisticated heir of (cultural; LZ) relativism'.

Happiness, Relations of Power and Cultural Studies

While postmodern anthropology reflects on the relations of power primarily in terms of the researcher's relationship towards the other peoples and cultures he or she is analyzing and interpreting, there is another field of research that prominently supplements the discussion about culture, happiness and power: cultural studies. Namely, while also reflecting on power in terms of the relationship between the researcher and his object of analysis (culture), the interdisciplinary field of cultural studies (see Barker 2002) predominately focuses on analyzing the workings of power within the object of analysis (culture) itself[12]. Insofar as they all share a similar conception of culture (see Hall 1999; Barker 2000, 2002), cultural studies is consonant with cultural psychology and the anthropology of well-being on the theory of cultural construction of happiness. Drawing from similar philosophical sources as postmodern anthropology, cultural studies does not share their problems with a thorough understanding of all the consequences of the cultural construction argument. More specifically, cultural studies is interested in examining the role and the consequences of power in relation to the social and the cultural construction of reality. In this sense, the cultural studies approach not only reflects 'on how hap-

[11] As we shall see, this conception of truth is very close to the Nietzschean and Foucauldian conceptions of truth.

[12] Regarding itself as a political project, cultural studies is also interested in changing and transforming those relations of power. As we shall argue, cultural studies should, therefore, also be interested in happiness in terms of their political project.

piness is represented within culture, but also on how happiness generates effects, bringing a certain world into existence' (Ahmed 2007/2008, p. 11).

According to cultural studies, cultural meanings and practices are never independent from the workings of power. Of course, the same holds for meanings and practices that enter in the cultural constitution of the experience of happiness and well-being, which includes two of their main components: the subject(s) of happiness/well-being and the conception(s)/notion(s) of happiness/well-being. The cultural construction of happiness is, thus, always closely connected with the relations of power in society. In other words, from the perspective of cultural studies, happiness is not only a result of a cultural constitution, but also a result of socially mediated relations of power linked to such a constitution: 'Cultural Studies might, in its very worldly orientation, offer a rigorous analysis of happiness and power: ideas of happiness support concepts of the good life that take the shape of some lives and not others' (Ahmed 2007/2008, p. 11). This means that what in a certain society and in a certain culture for most people counts as happiness always corresponds to a product of a particular historical constellation of relations between culture and power, through which a certain experience of happiness is constituted and established as dominant. For Ahmed (2007/2008, p. 11), critically reading happiness is, thus, 'a matter of reading how happiness and unhappiness are distributed and located within certain bodies and groups'.

Considering the workings of power in relation to happiness, we, therefore, cannot simply conceive of happiness and well-being as inherently positive and unproblematic cultural phenomena. Or, as stated by Ahmed (2007/2008, p. 7): 'Cultural studies can make an important contribution to debates about happiness precisely given its willingness to refuse to consent to its truth. We might even suspend belief that happiness is what we want, or that happiness is what is good'. In a critical mode, happiness has already been approached by Bruckner (2001), Binkley (2007), Ahmed et al. (2007/2008), Zevnik (2009) and Ahmed (2010), whose work we shall attempt to supplement in the following chapters.

Being critical towards happiness and not simply accepting it as an a priori positive notion and experience does not mean, however, that one has to take an a priori negative position towards happiness and well-being. Instead, it implies that we should reflect on the concepts and cultural workings of happiness and well-being as potentially problematic and dangerous. In this sense, we believe that the critical approach to happiness ought to follow Foucault (2000a, p. 256), who exclaimed, 'My point is not that everything is bad, but that everything is dangerous, which is not exactly the same as bad. If everything is dangerous, then we always have something to do. I think that the ethico-political choice we have to make every day is to determine which is the main danger'.

Following from this, we believe that besides (or better complementary with) a more negative/critical approach aiming to reflect on the possible dangerous aspects of the experience of happiness, the study of happiness (within cultural studies) should also involve a more positive approach to happiness understood in terms of a certain form of a general culture of the self. The first step in this direction has already been made by Barker (2002). Namely, arguing that the problems we face in the post-scarcity cultures 'are increasingly psychological, rather than material,' he proposed a new perspective/strategy in cultural studies concerned with emotions, spirituality, happiness and contentment. This book, however, will predominantly focus on the critical approach (for more on the positive approach to happiness in the context of cultural studies, see Barker 2000; Zevnik 2010).

In addition to the problematic (subtle) remains of ethnocentricity and the incomplete understanding of the cultural construction thesis inherent in anthropology of well-being and the cultural perspective, it could also be argued that the existent approaches in empirical happiness research are not conclusive enough in their historical analyses.

Happiness and History

The authors from within the cultural perspective rightly argue that the 'the history of the culture' is very important to the understanding of the contemporary experience of happiness (in Western culture) (Kitayama and Markus 2000; Lu and Gilmour 2004). At the same time, we have to note that attempts at historical analysis undertaken by the authors from the cultural perspective (see for e.g. Lu and Gilmour 2004) are still far from conveying comprehensive historical insights into the historical background of the Western experience of happiness and that anthropology of well-being and survey-based happiness research almost completely lack historical analysis.

There are at least two more detailed historical analyses of happiness available. As a philosopher, White (2006, p. viii) has written a *Brief History of Happiness* 'as it appears in Western philosophy,' in which he provides a historical overview of 'important philosophical problems in which the idea figures'. While White's history of happiness is limited to the realm of philosophy, McMahon (2006, p. xiv) has conceptualized his book as a broader 'intellectual history' of happiness: 'I do believe that a history of happiness, at least initially, should be an intellectual history, a history of conceptions of this perennial human end and the strategies devised to attain it, as these have evolved in different ethical, philosophical, religious, and, I would add, political contexts'.

While the intellectual history of happiness certainly forms an important part of any historical approach (to happiness), the work of the French historian and philosopher Michel Foucault (2001) has shown that a thorough in-depth historical analysis cannot be limited solely to the historical analysis of happiness 'as an idea' (McMahon 2006, p. xiv). In order to support his argument, Foucault (2001, p. 74) distinguishes between the 'history of ideas and the history of thought':

> Most of the time a historian of ideas tries to determine when a specific concept appears, and this moment is often identified by the appearance of a new word. But what I am attempting to do as a historian of thought is something different. I am trying to analyze the way institutions, practices, habits, and behavior become a problem for people who behave in specific sorts of ways, who have certain types of habits, who engage in certain kinds of practices,

> and who put to work specific kinds of institutions. The history of ideas involves the analysis of a notion from its birth, through its development, and in the setting of other ideas, which constitute its context. The history of thought is the analysis of the way an unproblematic field of experience, or a set of practices which were accepted without question, which were familiar and out of discussion, becomes a problem, raises discussion and debate, incites new reactions, and induces a crisis in the previously silent behavior, habits, practices, and institutions. The history of thought, understood in this way, is the history of the way people begin to take care of something, of the way they became anxious about this or that, for example, about madness, about crime, about sex, about themselves, or about truth.

The aim of history of thought, Foucault explains (2001, p. 171), is neither to analyze 'past people's behavior' nor 'ideas in their representative values,' but to analyze 'the process of "problematization"- which means: how and why certain things (behavior, phenomena, processes) became a problem'. More specifically: it is 'a matter of analyzing, not behaviors and ideas, nor societies and their "ideologies," but the problematizations through which being offers itself to be, necessarily, thought—and the practices on the basis of which these problematizations are formed' (Foucault 1990, p. 11). According to Foucault (1988, p. 257):

> Problematization doesn't mean representation of a preexisting object, nor the creation by discourse of an object that doesn't exist. It is the totality of discursive or non-discursive practices that introduces something into the play of true and false and constitutes it as an object for thought (whether in the form of moral reflection, scientific knowledge, political analysis, etc.) (Foucault 1988, p. 257).

In the case of happiness, this suggests an analysis of the problematization of happiness, which includes examining 'how and why were very different things in the world gathered together, characterized, analyzed, and treated' as happiness and 'what are the elements which are relevant' for the problematization of happiness (Foucault 2001, p. 171).

In addition to Foucault's critique of the traditional historical approach based on the difference between the history of ideas and the history of thought, he—inspired by Nietzsche—criticizes traditional history also on account of what he calls its 'suprahistorical perspective' (Foucault 2000b, p. 379). Namely, according to Foucault (2000b, p. 379), history in the traditional sense

> reintroduces (and always assumes) a suprahistorical perspective: a history whose function is to compose the finally reduced diversity of time into a totality fully closed upon itself; a history that always encourages subjective recognitions and attributes a form of reconciliation to all the displacements of the past; a history whose perspective on all that precedes it implies the end of time, a completed development. The historian's history finds its support outside of time and claims to base its judgments on an apocalyptic objectivity (Foucault 2000b, p. 379).

To claim such an 'apocalyptic objectivity,' Foucault explains (2000b, p. 379), a historical perspective has to maintain 'its belief in eternal truth, the immortality of the soul, and the nature of consciousness as always identical to itself'. When the historical sense is mastered by such a suprahistorical perspective, 'metaphysics can align it to the demands of objective science' (Foucault 2000b, p. 379).

The effect of such an objectifying suprahistorical perspective in traditional historical accounts of happiness such as White's and McMahon's is that by analyzing the "history of happiness" from antiquity to modern times, they essentially retrospectively project the idea and experience of happiness to periods in the history of Western culture when in fact those ideas didn't yet exist[13] or, better yet, when they were not yet problematized. In more concrete words, traditional historians of happiness assume that the ancient Greek Eudemonia, Roman Felicity or the medieval Christian idea of heaven are just variations of a universal and suprahistorical idea of happiness that, in essence, corresponds to basically the same thing. Or, as Bruckner (2010, p. 3) puts it, 'We are constantly projecting onto earlier periods or other cultures a conception and obsession that belongs solely to our own'.

Foucault (2000b, p. 379), on the other hand, argues that, even though we are inclined to 'believe that feelings are immutable,' in fact, 'every sentiment, particularly the noblest and most disinterested, has a history'. It, therefore, follows that we must record the historical 'singularity of events outside of any monotonous finality; it must seek them in the most unpromising places, in what we tend to feel is without history—in sentiments, love, conscience, instincts' (Foucault 2000b, p. 369); and, of course, in happiness.

In the Foucauldian perspective, the fact that happiness has a history, therefore, does not simply imply analysis of the historical evolution of happiness across various periods in the history of thought (i.e. in a suprahistorical sense) like that undertaken by White or McMahon. Rather, it implies that besides its cultural singularity, we also recognize its historical singularity. That is, strictly speaking, happiness is not only a characteristic solely of Western culture (as we have argued above), but it is also characteristic exclusive to a certain period in the history of Western culture (from the seventeenth century onwards to the present time, as our analysis in the following chapters will show). Of course, this doesn't mean that people in the past didn't have an ideal of existence, but rather that their experience connected to this ideal was so much different from our own modern experience of happiness that it is impossible to claim that we are dealing with the same thing. Furthermore, this also doesn't mean that the experiences from previous periods are not—at least to a certain extent—connected to each other. As we shall see, besides important discontinuities in the history of thought, there are often also certain continuities[14].

[13] We shall support this argument by an extensive analysis in the second part of the book.

[14] While the Foucauldian approach is often perceived as primarily focusing on discontinuities in the history of thought, that is not really the case. Foucault (1983) himself emphasized that the history of thought 'has nothing to do with continuity or discontinuity' because in history one 'can find either continuity or discontinuity'.

Chapter 3
The Return to Happiness: A New Interdisciplinary Approach to Happiness Research

Critical discussion in the Chap. 2 has indicated that the existent approaches within the field of empirical happiness research mostly fail in providing adequate critical accounts of happiness in relation to culture. The philosophy of well-being and quantitative survey-based cross-cultural happiness/well-being research articulate or assume universal notions and definitions of well-being that are problematic on account of their ethnocentrism. In addition, the quantitative cross-cultural well-being research has proven to be limited and incomplete.

The recent approaches in empirical happiness research from the cultural perspective and anthropology of well-being in many respects productively criticize and complement the survey-based approaches, arguing that happiness and well-being are not universal, but rather culturally and historically specific social constructions. In addition, they have introduced an array of new (mostly qualitative) research methods, which are more inclusive in mapping out the cultural contours of happiness. However, we have also pointed out some problematic—mostly theoretical—issues and lacunae with the cultural perspective and anthropology of well-being approaches that were illuminated with the help of postmodern anthropology and cultural studies. Namely, in order for these approaches to be able to discover differences in cultural construction of well-being across cultures, they also have to implicitly or explicitly articulate certain universal criteria for what counts as a cultural construction of well-being, which, strictly speaking, can also be ethnocentric. We have noted that these problems persist as part of a larger issue, which is that they both fail to acknowledge all the consequences of the cultural construction thesis and apply them to the research on happiness and well-being. In order to tackle this issue, we have drawn from postmodern anthropology and cultural studies that understand the cultural construction thesis not only on the methodological level (as do anthropology of well-being and cultural perspective in happiness studies), but also on the levels of epistemology, ontology, ethics and relations of power.

We are on the same page as postmodern anthropology, which, with the help of philosophers like Rorty and Foucault, contravenes modern epistemology and the scientific method that is based on it. This implies refusing the possibility of any universal and objective knowledge and notions about the world and instead adopting anti-representationalism, anti-foundationalism and positionalism. Applying these

L. Zevnik, *Critical Perspectives in Happiness Research*,
DOI 10.1007/978-3-319-04403-3_3, © Springer International Publishing Switzerland 2014

notions to the research and study of happiness and well-being means refusing all universal notions of well-being and happiness, even the ones that constitute the ground, in order to discover differences in cultural constructions of happiness and well-being assumed by anthropology and the cultural perspective in empirical happiness research. Insofar as well-being and happiness are notions and experiences specific to Western culture, we therefore have to analyze them precisely as that: as singular cultural phenomena that have only emerged within Western culture in a particular time period. This "return to happiness"—as we have called it—implies that we have to analyze happiness as a culturally and historically singular experience in Western culture that is constituted by specific cultural meanings and practices. As a consequence the book intentionally does not provide an a priori universal definition of happiness but rather traces the unfolding of wider social and mundane processes in which happiness is defined (and made meaningful) by individuals, groups of individuals and social institutions. In this sense it could be argued that the definition of happiness spans across the whole book and is not limited to a condensed technical definition plagued by the danger of ethnocentrism.

Taking the notion of positionality into account, we also have to acknowledge that we cannot produce knowledge that would objectively represent happiness and well-being in Western culture. Instead, we can only produce what Clifford (1986) and Foucault (2002) call a serious, true fiction about the meanings and practices constituting the experience of happiness in Western culture.

With the help of postmodern anthropology and especially cultural studies, we have also pointed out that the existent approaches of empirical happiness research ignore the workings of power in relation to the cultural construction of happiness. In this sense, the perspectives of cultural studies and postmodern anthropology encourage us to also examine the cultural processes, which caused a particular conception and experience of happiness to become dominant, the relations of power involved in that process and the effects of that conception and experience for individuals and society. Such a critical analysis of the experience of happiness in Western culture also has to include a critical reflection of "scientific" research on happiness and well-being, which—as we shall argue—also plays an important role in the cultural constitution of a dominant regime of happiness. In this sense, we certainly agree with Foucault (1988, p. 106), who maintained that science is a way of exercising power: 'the fact that societies can become the object of scientific observation, that human behavior became, from a certain point on, a problem to be analyzed and resolved, all that is bound up, I believe with the mechanism of power—which, in a given moment, indeed analyzed that object (society, man, etc.) and presented it as a problem to be resolved' (Foucault 1988, p. 106). As a consequence, we believe that well-being research and philosophy of well-being focusing either on Western culture or other cultures also have to be put in the cultural and historical context of the Western experience of happiness and critically dissected. Researching and studying happiness and well-being, then, should not only aim to explain the construction of happiness and well-being in everyday life, but also to (self)-critically examine how research, measurement, scientific and philosophical notions of well-being and happiness have become constituted and how they are connected to the dominant mode of experience of happiness in Western culture. This must include critically examining what is their historical substratum; how and why the problem of measuring and researching happiness has emerged in the history of Western culture; what are its aims, strategies and mechanisms; what is their role in the interplay of power relations and what are its effects. All of these issues also need to be taken into account with the emerging field of neuroscience of happiness that promises importand new empirical insights into the topic of happiness.

Last but not least, we have argued that the existent historical analysis of happiness, which is vital to a thorough understanding of its specifics, has so far been inadequate, mostly focusing only on the intellectual history and ignoring what Foucault calls the history of thought. In addition, they also employ a problematic suprahistorical perspective.

Towards a New Interdisciplinary Approach to the Study of Happiness

We have argued in our discussion above that besides having certain ethnocentric and theoretical issues, the existent approaches in the empirical happiness and well-being research do not provide a sufficient theoretical and methodological framework to address all the aspects that we had identified as important for a critical understanding of the cultural and historical constitution of happiness in Western culture. As a consequence, we shall attempt to develop our own approach for the critical analysis of happiness in Western culture, which will be based on postmodern anthropology and cultural studies. More specifically, we shall mostly draw from the approach developed by Michel Foucault, which, although occupying an important position in both (postmodern) anthropology and cultural studies, hasn't yet been used to formulate a holistic critical perspective on happiness. In our view, the choice of the Foucauldian nominalist approach is relevant because it enables us to examine happiness as an experience in all the aspects our analysis above has shown to be vital for the critical understanding of this phenomenon in Western culture. Namely, the Foucauldian approach firstly implies

> a systematic skepticism toward all anthropological universals—which does not mean rejecting them all from the start, outright and once and for all, but that nothing of that order must be accepted that is not strictly indispensable. In regard to human nature or the categories that may be applied to the subject, everything in our knowledge which is suggested to us as being universally valid must be tested and analyzed (Foucault 2000b, p. 461).

This enables us to articulate a methodological framework that does not assume any a priori universal notions of happiness and well-being. Foucault (2002, p. 226) also calls the procedure of analysis that circumvents the anthropological universals "eventualization," which 'means making visible a singularity at places where there is a temptation to invoke a historical constant, an immediate anthropological trait, or an obviousness that imposes itself uniformly on all. To show that things "weren't as necessary as all that,". Foucault explains eventualization with the help of examples from his research: 'It wasn't as a matter of course that mad people came to be regarded as mentally ill; it wasn't self-evident that the only thing to be done with a criminal was to lock him up'. With the help of Ahmed (2007, 2008, p. 9), we can add that it certainly also wasn't self-evident 'that there is something called happiness; that happiness is good; and that happiness can be known and measured' (Ahmed 2007, 2008, p. 9). The next step of eventualization enables us to rediscover 'the connections, encounters, supports, blockages, plays of forces, strategies, and so on, that at a given moment establish what subsequently counts as being self-evident, universal, and necessary' (Foucault 2000b, p. 227). In our case, how has happiness become something so self-evident, universal and central in Western culture?

In addition, the Foucauldian approach refuses modern epistemology and thoroughly adopts the positions of anti-representationalism, anti-foundationalism and positionality, which are not adopted only when analyzing the present, but also to the realm of historical analysis. In this sense, it not only enables us to critically examine notions and experiences of happiness and well-being as cultural constructs, but also 'as historical constructs' (Foucault 2000b, p. 462). We have already seen above that a Foucauldian history of thought aimed at analyzing 'historicity of forms of experience' (Foucault 2000a, p. 200) provides the tools for a more thorough historical analysis of the experience of happiness in Western culture than the history of ideas. In this sense, it enables us to examine the cultural and historical constitution of both major components of the experience of happiness: the notions of happiness and the subject of happiness. More specifically, it enables us to examine the process by which notions of happiness and well-being have become constituted in Western culture and the process by which the subject of happiness has become constituted in Western culture. Moreover, it can also explain more thoroughly the relationship between the concepts of the subject/self of happiness and the experience of happiness that hasn't yet been explored by the existent approaches in happiness studies. And last but not least, considering that Foucault has put forward one of the most innovative and complex analyses of power, his method enables us to critically reflect on all the aspects of happiness mentioned above in terms of their connectedness with the relations of power.

Before we can apply the Foucauldian perspective to the study of happiness, we must first look more closely at its main theoretical and methodological stakes.

The Specifics of the Foucauldian Approach

When speaking of philosopher Michel Foucault, who once said, 'Do not ask me who I am and do not ask me to remain the same' (2004, p. 19), we should always remember that we are actually speaking about multiple Foucaults. Furthermore, insofar as Foucault's life was strongly influenced by his philosophical work—and vice versa—there are not only multiple Foucaults, but also multiple stages of Foucault's work, each having its own particular methodology, categorical apparatus and philosophical insights. All this is related to the fact that Foucault never intended to formulate a general and unified philosophical system, but rather explored particular transformations of specific problems within his subjective historical experience: 'I am an experimenter and not a theorist. I call a theorist someone who constructs a general system, either deductive or analytical, and applies it to different fields in a uniform way. That isn't my case. I'm an experimenter in the sense that I write in order to change myself and in order not to think the same thing as before' (Foucault 2002, p. 240).

Foucault hoped to achieve these transformations with the help of critical reflections upon problems within his/our historical experience. In this sense, his philosophy was—even when providing broader philosophical insights—always grounded in the analysis of concrete fields of experience. In his words, the main imperative of his work was to 'never lose sight of the reference of a concrete example that may serve as a ground for the analysis' (Foucault 2000a, p. 7). As a consequence, Foucault's methodology was in constant development, enabling him to explore the specifics of every particular problem he had been analyzing. As such, every instance of "Foucault's" methodological grip was just as much a tool for a particular analysis as it had also been its end result: 'When I begin a book, not only do I not know what I'll be thinking at the end, but it's not very clear to me what method I will employ. Each of my books is a way of carving out an object and of fabricating a method of analysis' (Foucault 2000b, p. 240).

Foucault's philosophical insights and reflections as well as his methodological approach were, hence, never final or closed. Rather, they were characterized by a constant experimental openness, maintaining a reflective horizon always open for possible methodological and analytical reevaluation and development:

> I wouldn't want what I may have said or written to be seen as laying any claims to totality. I don't try to universalize what I say; conversely, what I don't say isn't meant to be thereby disqualified as being of no importance. My work takes place between unfinished abutments and anticipatory strings of dots. I like to open up a space of research, try it out, and then if it doesn't work, try again somewhere else. On many points—I am thinking especially of the relations between dialectics, genealogy, and strategy—I am still working and don't yet know whether I am going to get anywhere. What I say ought to be taken as "propositions," "game openings" where those who may be interested are invited to join in—they are not meant as dogmatic assertions that have to be taken or left en bloc. My books aren't treatises in philosophy or studies of history: at most, they are philosophical fragments put to work in a historical field of problems (Foucault 2002, p. 223).

A similar openness also marks Foucault's relation to transformative practice (of writing books): 'it would probably not be worth the trouble of making books if they failed to teach the author something he had not known before, if they did not lead to unforeseen places, and if they did not disperse one toward a strange and new relation with himself. The pain and pleasure of the book is to be an experience'[1] (Foucault 2000a, p. 205).

---

[1] In this sense, Foucault was writing what he called experience books (fr. *livre experience*). In order to understand what he meant exactly by experience books, we have to consider that the French word experience not only refers to experience, but also to the word experiment. An experience

Foucault's specific philosophical approach does not mean that he left the plethora of his singular accounts and problematizations completely methodologically disconnected, and the broader philosophical conclusions that could be drawn out of them, unarticulated. Even though his ideas and methodology evolved and transformed considerably along his philosophical trajectory, often producing radical theoretical breaks, he refused to completely discard his previous methodology and philosophical insights. Rather, he tried to remold and reposition them so that they would serve his current research and fit into his latest line of work. As a consequence, in many of his interviews and shorter texts he reflected back on his previous research and insights in order to reassess, reorganize and synthesize them, thus connecting them with his current and future line of thought: 'They are (the shorter texts L.Z.) something like a scaffolding that serves as a link between a work that is coming to an end and another one that's about to begin' and, as such, help 'to define another possible project' (Foucault 2002, p. 240). In shorter texts and interviews, Foucault also illuminates and reflects on the contours of the vibrant shifts in his thought[2] and constantly provides meta re-readings and clarifications of his previous works that enabled him to draw broader philosophical insights. Following from this, the complexity and inclusiveness of Foucault's methodology and theoretical apparatus increased with the number and the nature of the problems he had queried. Foucault's deeper and more profound analysis of any field of experience published in his books, hence, always strived to produce the critical reflection of that particular problem, the methodological tools and categorical apparatus developed to provide that reflection and the transformations of his own thought and potentially also the thought of his readers related to that problem (2002, pp. 239–297).

When speaking of Michel Foucault, it is not only the multiple stages of his work that one has to consider, but also multiple layers of his philosophical project, which are all closely interconnected. First, Foucault is a certain mode of critical philosophical attitude/reflection; second, Foucault is an open/fluid categorical apparatus and methodology; and, third, Foucault also provides philosophical insights into the problems he had analyzed. This means that in order to better understand Foucault's specific philosophical project, one has to always try to read and analyze it as a whole; that is, to approach any segment of his work in the context of his entire oeuvre and at the same time also consider his philosophical attitude and the characteristic aims of his philosophical project.

In this sense, Foucault's late(-er) texts especially are extremely important, as they are obviously the most complex and inclusive, both in terms of methodology as well as in terms of philosophical apparatus and insights. Moreover, in them, Foucault also provides clear signals on how to reinterpret and use his entire opus. Agreeing with Davidson (1986, p. 221) that 'Foucault is usually his own best interpreter,' we, thus, believe that one can benefit greatly from approaching Foucault's

book for Foucault is, thus, meant to produce an experience that is at the same time an experiment undertaken by the author himself (and to which his readers are also invited).

[2] In the following, we shall see that there are roughly four major theoretical shifts in Foucault's work.

philosophy and methodology not only in a linear fashion from his early to his late work, but also in retrograde: dynamically re-assessing every segment of his oeuvre in a way Foucault re-interpreted it in his later texts.

With such a holistic view on Foucault, we are not implying, however, that we have to look for the "real" or "ultimate" Foucault. In claiming that Foucault is his own best interpreter, we are also not implying that we should blindly follow his thought and refuse to depart from what he says. Rather, we wish to stress that by failing to see the specifics of Foucault's unconventional approach to philosophy in a broader sense, we are running the risk of losing the complexity and subtle nuances of his insights.

Taking the specifics of Foucault's philosophical project into account, it is, thus, problematic to consider Foucault's work solely as an object of theoretical analysis and, hence, focus predominantly on his categorical apparatus and philosophical insights. It is also not entirely appropriate to approach him as an (philosophical) author in a conventional sense. As a matter of fact, with his problematization of the concept, Foucault (2000b, pp. 205–223) himself implicitly alluded that his work should be approached somewhat differently. That is, insofar as Foucault never wanted to be a philosopher in a conventional modern sense of the word, nor did he intend to articulate a philosophical system, it is not very fitting to solely evaluate him in such terms. This would inevitably mean superimposing certain standards upon a thinker who tried to work in a completely different framework with completely different aims.

Even though a strictly philosophical approach to Foucault's work is relevant to some extent, it also runs the risk of losing the main trajectory of Foucault's project, which was to reflect on mundane fields of human life in order to induce certain transformations of experience. Insofar as Foucault's insights were always founded on concrete analyses of certain problems within our historical experience that aimed to induce certain concrete effects for our experience, I believe that taking a Foucauldian position is first and foremost about taking a certain critical attitude towards our present experience and towards ourselves. This means trying to apply Foucauldian methodology to new problems within our historical experience rather than only accepting his philosophical insights or engaging in philosophical discussions regarding his work. Insofar as Foucault himself developed his philosophical insights with the help of 'concrete examples that may serve as a ground for the analysis' (Foucault 2000a, p. 7), new applications of Foucauldian methodology can, thus, also play an important part in the further development of Foucauldian theory itself. The field of the so-called Governmentality Studies (see Burchell et al. 1991) is a very good example of how Foucauldian theory is much more vibrant if it is also developed by critically applying it to new fields of experience rather than only relying on abstract philosophical readings and comparative analysis.

If one aims at applying Foucauldian methodology to a particular phenomena/problem/field of research, which of the multiple segments of Foucault's work is one to use then? The most common strategy would be to select the methodology and philosophical apparatus developed by Foucault when analyzing a problem similar to one's own field of interest. Another even simpler one would be to arbitrarily use any particular segment of Foucault's thought, which appears most suitable. In our view, however, one should be extremely careful with such simple strategies because—as we have argued above—the complexity and inclusiveness of Foucault's methodology and theoretical apparatus increased with the number and the nature of the problems he had queried.

Following from this, we shall first try to approach the main aspects of Foucault's work with which we will attempt to formulate a methodology that could be used for analysis of phenomena within our historical experience. Here, we have to note that by this we do not intend to build something like a closed system of Foucault's philosophy, as this would obviously run contrary to the essential spirit of Foucault's philosophical approach. Rather, our primary aim is to encompass the broadest explanatory and transformational potential of Foucault's work taken as a whole. Of course, this also does not mean uncritically adopting Foucault's methodology and philosophical insights, for this would be against the critical attitude we are trying to pursue. The aim of this second part is to articulate a Foucauldian-inspired methodological point of departure that will then be further developed and critically revised by applying it to a new field of research—happiness in Western culture.

In the spirit of the Foucauldian approach, we will attempt to approach the analysis of happiness as an experience 'that one comes out transformed' (Foucault 2002, p. 239), which hopefully will also 'have a certain value for others, so that the experience is available for others to have' (Foucault 2002, p. 244). To that end, I will first examine the broadest philosophical foundations of Foucault's approach.

Foucauldian Subject and Experience

Foucault did the bulk of his "meta-theoretical" work towards the end of his life. Reflecting on Kant's philosophical project and especially on his answer to the question *What is enlightenment?* (Kant 2009), Foucault outlined the broadest philosophical foundations of his work. Kant's quite obscure text on the enlightenment published in *Berlinische Monatshrift* in 1784 seems important to Foucault (1988, p. 86), especially because it 'introduces a new type of question into the field of philosophical reflection': 'What is our present? What is the present field of possible experiences' (Foucault 1988, p. 95)? 'What is our actuality? What are we as part of this actuality' (Foucault 1983)? Foucault (1988, p. 95) believes that the introduction of such philosophical reflection means that Kant has 'founded the two great critical traditions between which modern philosophy is divided'. The first is the 'tradition of philosophy that poses the question of the conditions in which true knowledge is possible' (Foucault 1988, p. 95). Foucault (1988, p. 95) further explains that 'on that basis, it may be said that a whole stretch of modern philosophy from the nineteenth century has been presented, developed as the analytics of truth'. There is, however, another method of critical interrogation in modern philosophy. Foucault (1988, p. 95) sees it emerging precisely in Kant's texts on the Enlightenment: 'one may opt for a critical philosophy of truth in general, or one may opt for a critical thought that will take the form of an ontology of ourselves, an ontology of the present; it is this form of philosophy that, from Hegel, through Nietzsche and Max Weber, to the Frankfurt school has founded a form of reflection in which I have tried to work'. Following this critical tradition, Foucault concludes (2002, p. 336), implies that 'maybe the most certain of all philosophical problems is the problem of the present time, and of what we are, in this very moment'. This statement by Foucault already alludes to the field of our actuality that in Foucault's view requires the most of our critical attention: the subject.

Such a critical philosophical approach is relevant to the critical analysis of happiness because happiness represents an important part of our present field of experiences/actuality and, thus, must be critically examined. This implies conducting a critical ontology of happiness in Western culture, which has to include critical ontologies of the experience of happiness and the subject of happiness (which are—as we shall see—closely connected). As we shall argue towards the end of this second part of the book, a critical ontology can be conducted through the genealogical approach and archeological method.

Reading only Foucault's major books, one could conclude that while the earlier Foucault completely refused the concept of the subject, the later Foucault suddenly reanimated and rehabilitated the subject. However, in one of his last interviews reflecting back on his entire philosophical opus, Foucault clearly stated that from the beginning the main objective of his work was actually to 'create a history of the different modes by which, in our culture, human beings are made subjects' (Foucault 2002, p. 326). By closely examining Foucault's approach, we can see that what he indeed refused throughout his work (and after all what he actually meant by talking about the death of man) was not the notion of the subject as such, but a priori theories of the subject that perceive the subject as a substance. According to Foucault, refusing the subject actually means 'that there is no sovereign, founding subject, a universal form of subject to be found everywhere' (Foucault 1988, p. 50). In this sense, subject is not a substance, but 'it is a form' (Foucault 2000a, p. 290):

> and this form is not primarily or always identical to itself. You do not have the same type of relationship to yourself when you constitute yourself as a political subject who goes to vote or speaks at a meeting and when you are seeking to fulfill your desires in a sexual relationship. Undoubtedly there are relationships and interferences between these different forms of the subject; but we are not dealing with the same type of subject. In each case, one plays, one establishes a different type of relationship to oneself.

In his understanding of the subject, Foucault was following Nietzsche who argued against the Western metaphysics that, according to him, maintained a notion of an ahistorical and universal subject as the foundation of all knowledge and experience of man and the world. For Nietzsche (1968, num. 485), '"the subject" is the fiction that many similar states in us are the effect of one substratum':

> A quantum of force is equivalent to a quantum of drive, will, effect—more, it is nothing other than this very driving, willing, effecting and only owing to the seduction of language (and the fundamental errors of reason which are petrified in it) that conceives and misconceives all effects as conditioned by something that causes, by a "subject," can it appear otherwise. For just as the popular mind separates the lightning from its flash and takes the

> latter for an action, for the operation of a subject called lightning, so popular morality also separates strength from expressions of strength, as if there were a neutral substratum behind the strong man, which was free to express strength or not to do so. But there is no such substratum; there is no 'being' behind doing, effecting, becoming; the "doer" is merely a fiction added to the deed—the deed is everything (Nietzsche 1989, num. 13).

Inspired by Nietzsche, Foucault attempted to provide an alternative to a modern philosophical tradition from Descartes and Kant to Husserl and Sartre[3], which he called 'the philosophy of the subject' (Foucault 1999, p. 159). For Foucault (2000a, p. 290), the philosophy of the subject started 'out with the theory of the subject,' and based on this theory asked 'how a given form of knowledge was possible'. As a consequence, this kind of philosophy sees 'the foundation of all knowledge and the principle of all signification as steaming from the meaningful subject' (Foucault 1999, p. 159). The fact that from the beginning Foucault was rejecting a conception of the subject as an unchangeable and fixed foundation does not mean that he was not interested in it. On the contrary, this was exactly why he tried 'to show how the subject constituted itself, in one specific form or another/.../through certain practices that were also games of truth, practices of power, and so on' (Foucault 2000a, p. 290). The fact that Foucault refused a priori theories of the subject was precisely the reason why he was interested in it in terms of illuminating its constant dynamic historical constitution: 'one has to dispense with the constituent subject, to get rid of the subject itself, that's to say to arrive at an analysis that can account for the constitution of the subject within a historical framework' (Foucault 2002, p. 118). Foucault (1999, p. 160), thus, 'tried to get out from the philosophy of the subject through a genealogy of this subject, by studying the constitution of the subject across history which has led us up to the modern concept of the self'.

Foucault is interested in a historical analysis of the constitution of the subject because he maintains—again following Nietzsche—that the subject is not only singular, but also radically historical:

> Currently when one does history—the history of ideas, of knowledge, or simply history—one sticks to this subject of knowledge, to this subject of representation as the point of origin from which knowledge is possible and truth appears. It would be interesting to try to see how a subject came to be constituted that is not definitely given, that is not the thing on the bases of which truth happens to history—rather, a subject that constitutes itself within history and is constantly established and re-established by history. It is toward that radical critique of the human subject by history that we should direct our efforts (Foucault 2002, p. 3).

Insofar as 'the self is nothing than the correlate of technology built into our history' (Foucault 1999, p. 181), the task then 'is to expose a body totally imprinted by history,' which 'inscribes itself in the nervous system, in temperament, in the digestive apparatus; it appears in faulty respiration, in improper diets, in the debilitated and prostrate bodies of those whose antecessors committed errors' (Foucault 2000b, p. 375). The subject indeed is form rather than substance (Foucault 2000a, p. 290) and, as such, a result of the intersection of 'fluid, historically constituted

[3] In one of his interviews, Foucault (2000b, pp. 433–459) explained that in this sense he was a part of a new philosophical current in France in the 1960s and 1970s, which stressed providing an alternative to the prevalent phenomenological approach and its theories of the subject that were common in France at the time.

and constantly transformed relations to the self' (Gros 2005, p. 526) and various techniques of domination. Gros (2005, p. 526) further clarifies Foucault's notion of a historical subject, which is inevitably tied to the effects of power: 'the individual subject only ever emerges at the intersection of a technique of domination and techniques of the self. It is the fold of processes of subjectivation over procedures of subjection, according to more or less overlapping linings subject to history'.

Such understanding of the subject implies and enables an examination of different modes by which, in the history of Western culture, human beings have been constituted as subjects of happiness. However, in order to comprehend how, according to Foucault, individuals are historically constituted as subjects (of happiness), we first have to explore how he understands the relationship between subject and experience.

The Relationship Between Subject and Experience

According to Foucault (1988, p. 253), the subject is not the condition of possibility of experience. On the contrary, 'It is experience which is the rationalization of a process, itself provisional, which results in a subject, or rather in subjects[4]. I will call subjectivation the procedure by which one obtains the constitution of a subject or, more precisely, of subjectivity, which is, of course, only one of the given possibilities of organization of a self-consciousness' (Foucault 1988, p. 253).

Taking the historical constitution of subjects into account, Foucault's aim was, therefore, to 'consider the very historicity of forms of experience' (Foucault 2000a, p. 200), where 'the formation, development, and transformation of forms of experience' can be situated in the domain of 'a history of thought'[5] (Foucault 2000a, p. 200). According to Foucault (2002, p. 403), the aim of history of thought was 'the historical analysis of the relationships between our thought and our practices':

> "Thought," understood in this way, then, is not to be sought only in theoretical formulations such as those of philosophy and science; it can and must be analyzed in every manner of speaking, doing, or behaving in which the individual appears and acts as a knowing subject, as an ethical or juridical subject, as a subject conscious of himself and others. In this sense, thought is understood as the very form of action—as action insofar as it implies the play of true and false, the acceptance or refusal of rules, the relation to oneself and others. The study of forms of experience can, thus, proceed from an analysis of "practices"—discursive or not—as long as one qualifies that word to mean the different systems of action insofar as they are inhabited by thought as I have characterized it here.

Even though the notion of experience plays an important role[6] in Foucault's philosophical opus, he never provided an explicit definition. According to O'Leary

[4] Following from this, Foucault (1990, p. 6) also described his philosophical project as 'an analysis of the "games of truth," the games of truth and error through which being is historically constituted as experience'.

[5] Foucault held a chair with the same title at the famous College de France.

[6] In this regard we tend to agree with O'Leary (2010, p. 181) who argues that 'Foucault's work, almost in its entirety, can be read as a contribution to a fully historicized philosophy of experience'.

(2008), following Foucault's somewhat scattered uses of the term in different contexts along the arch of his theoretical development, it is nevertheless possible to map out the evolution and the scope of Foucault's concept of experience, which is central to the understanding of the historical constitution of subjects.

In *History of Madness* (2006), first published in 1964, Foucault described experience as 'everything that could be felt and formulated about madness at the beginning of the Renaissance'. In the same book, Foucault further argues that the practice of internment at least partly illuminates 'the mode in which madness was perceived, and lived, by the classical age'. Following from this is that the 'the first aspect of any experience, then, will be the forms of perception or sensibility which it makes possible—or even necessary. A given structure of experience makes possible and gives rise to certain ways of sensing, seeing, feeling an object' (O'Leary 2008, p. 9). In other words, experience for Foucault 'involves the way in which a given object is seen and conceptualized in a given culture' (O'Leary 2008, p. 9) during a certain time.

However, as O'Leary further explains (2008, p. 9), for Foucault 'these forms of experience are not the only components of a structure of experience'. Namely, in *History of Madness*, Foucault (2006) also argues that besides being a form of sensibility, the experience of madness also 'comprises both the institutional practices of internment and the forms of knowledge which develop within and bolster those institutions' (O'Leary 2008, p. 9). This opens up the domain, which Foucault (2000a) would later call the power/knowledge (truth) axis of any form of experience. Foucault used the second aspect of experience also in the *Order of things* (1994), where he explained that his aim was to illuminate the 'experience of order' between the sixteenth and nineteenth centuries. More specifically, how was 'the experience of language'—a 'global and cultural experience' of the late Renaissance transformed into a new form of experience in classical age? The second aspect of experience of any kind of phenomena would then include the forms of consciousness, sensibility, practical engagement and (scientific) knowledge, which take those particular phenomena as their object.

While in his earlier writing (early 1960s) Foucault used the concept of experience quite often, O'Leary observes 'that after the late 1960s, and up until the late 1970s, he was less and less willing to characterize his work in terms of investigation of experience' (O'Leary 2008, p. 10). O'Leary (2008, p. 10) believes that 'this was a result of his increasing dissatisfaction with the fluidity of the concept, but also of the fact that the concept, with its connotations of individual psychology, clashed with his new focus on bodies, resistance and power'. In that period, Foucault was also most explicit in his critique of the general, universal subject (mentioned above), which culminated in *Archeology of Knowledge* (2004). As a consequence, in *Archeology* he was somewhat skeptical about the way in which he used the notion of experience in the History of Madness because he believed that it carried the danger of re-introducing 'an anonymous and general subject of history' (Foucault 2004).

However, with Foucault's third and last major theoretical turn in the late 1970s, the notion of experience had returned. In the preface to History of Sexuality, vol. 2, for example, Foucault (1990, p. 199) explained that his 'object was to analyze sexuality as a historically singular form of experience'. Inspired by his research in sexuality and the modes of subjectivities in antiquity, Foucault found a way to re-conceptualize the notion of experience without the danger of re-introducing a general and universal subject. The notion of experience is now used by Foucault 'to indicate the general forms of thought, perception, and practice that characterize a particular area of human life during a particular historical period' (O'Leary 2010, p. 165). The mode of the constitution of the subject of any object (e.g. the subject of madness) would now include three closely connected domains/axes of experience, each representing a particular stage of his work. In the extended version of the preface to HS2, Foucault describes his three theoretical shifts, which reveal the main stages of his work.

> A theoretical shift had seemed necessary in order to analyze what was often designated as the advancement of learning; it led me to examine the forms of discursive practices that articulated the human sciences. A theoretical shift had also been required in order to analyze what is often described as the manifestations of "power"; it led me to examine, rather, the manifold relations, the open strategies, and the rational techniques that articulate the exercise of powers. It appeared that I now had to undertake a third shift, in order to analyze what is termed "the subject." It seemed appropriate to look for the forms and modalities of the relation to self by which the individual constitutes and recognizes himself qua subject (Foucault 1990, p. 6).

Using a broader conception of experience, Foucault (2000a, pp. 202–205) joined all four stages of his work, which earlier may have seemed like a series of disconnected modes of inquiry, into a more coherent, holistic and inclusive methodological framework:

> I tried to locate three major types of problems: the problem of truth, the problem of power, and the problem of individual conduct. These three domains of experience can only be understood in relation to each other, not independently. What bothered me about the previous books is that I considered the first two experiences without taking the third one into account. By bringing to light this third experience, it seemed to provide a kind of guiding thread which, in order to justify itself, did not need to resort to somewhat rhetorical methods of avoiding one of the three fundamental domains of experience (Foucault 1988, p. 243).

A critical reflection of any object (like madness, sexuality or, in our case, happiness), therefore, needs to address the axis of truth around it (roughly corresponding to his work in the 1960s like *Archeology of Knowledge and The Order of Things*; the relations of power connected to it by which certain individuals or groups of individuals try to control the conduct of others (roughly corresponding to his work in the 1970s like Discipline and Punish); and last but not least the relationship individuals establish with themselves while relating to that object—rapport a soi/ethics (this domain was elucidated by Foucault especially in the last two volumes of History of Sexuality).

All three domains/axes of experience have the following characteristics: they have a history (Foucault 2000a); they are tightly interweaved and 'these three domains of experience can only be understood one in relation to the others and cannot be understood one without the others' (Foucault 1988, p. 243); they have 'no chronological hierarchy' (O'Leary 2008, p. 11) and 'the relative importance of these three axes is not always the same for all forms of experience' (Foucault 2000, p. 202). In the case of Foucault's notion of experience, we can again observe the same specific pattern of his philosophical development, which we had already noted above, in the introduction to this part. That is, the evolution of Foucault's notion of experience can hardly be understood as a simple cumulative process, but rather as a complex synergic process: 'Indeed,' O'Leary explains (2008, p. 11), if the second phase does not so much add power to knowledge as introduce a new concept—power-knowledge—we could say that the final phase introduces another new concept—power-knowledge-to the self'[7].

Insofar as the concept of experience enables the late Foucault to effectively conjoin virtually all the major lines of enquiry undertaken throughout his entire oeuvre hence producing a strong analytical tool for the reflection of our actuality, we agree with O'Leary (2010), who argues that Foucault can be very productively read as a philosopher of experience. In the following, we shall use Foucault's understanding of experience as a methodological framework for the analysis of happiness in Western culture.

Before we look more closely at each of the domains of experience, we have to note that Foucault's main concepts of truth, power and relation to the self changed and developed considerably during the course of his philosophical development. As a consequence, it is difficult to talk about any of them in a unified sense. Since we are not conducting a purely theoretical analysis, we will not engage in a very detailed historical overview of the respective concepts in Foucault's thought. Instead, we will focus primarily on Foucault's most recent conception of each of the axes (which includes insights from his earlier conceptions anyway) and place more emphasis on their potential to be applied to concrete areas of research. We have argued that the three domains/axes of experience are always closely correlated. For the sake of clarity, we will begin by describing the axis of power and then explore how it connects to the axis of truth and the axis of relationship to the self. Finally, we will explore two main modes in which all three axes of experience connect to each other, transforming individuals into a particular type of subject.

In the following chapters, we shall then use the three-axis in order to analyze how the subject and the experience of happiness are constituted in Western culture.

Power (Relations)

Foucault aimed to provide an alternative to juridical theories of power based on legal models and sovereignty common to both liberalism and Marxism: 'What we need, however, is a political philosophy that isn't erected around the problem of sovereignty or, therefore, around the problems of law and prohibition. We need to cut off

[7] Taking the openness of the Foucauldian approach into account, we have to add that the three axes identified by Foucault should not be taken as the final domains of possible experience. With further analysis, perhaps a new axis of experience could be discovered.

the King's head: in political theory that has still to be done' (Foucault 2002, p. 122). In Foucault's (2002, p. 327) view, it was 'necessary to expand the dimensions of a definition of power if one wanted to use this definition in studying the objectivizing of the subject'. Rejecting juridical conceptions of power, Foucault (1978, p. 92) conceives power neither in terms of 'a group of institutions and mechanisms that ensure the subservience of the citizens of a given state' nor in terms of 'a mode of subjugation which, in contrast to violence, has the form of the rule'. Namely, according to Foucault (2002, p. 342), an attempt to analyze 'power relations as one finds them in certain closed institutions' presents the following problems:

- the fact that an important part of the mechanisms put into operation by an institution are designed to ensure its own preservation brings with it the risk of deciphering functions that are essentially reproductive, especially in power relations within institutions
- in analyzing power relations from the standpoint of institutions, one lays oneself open to seeking the explanation and the origin of the former in the latter, that is to say in sum, to explain power by power
- insofar as institutions act essentially by bringing into play two elements, explicit or tacit regulations and an apparatus, one risks giving to one or the other an exaggerated privilege in the relations of power and, hence, seeing in the latter only modulations of law and coercion

This, however, Foucault warns (2002, p. 343), 'is not to deny the importance of institutions in the establishment of power relations, but rather to suggest that one must analyze institutions from the standpoint of power relations rather than vice versa, and that the fundamental point of anchorage of the relationships, even if they are embodied and crystallized in an institution, is to be found outside the institution'. Moreover, power is also not a general system of domination exerted by one group over another (Foucault 1978, p. 92). That is, contrary to common understandings, for Foucault (2000a, p. 291) power cannot be conceived simply as 'a political structure, a government, a dominant social class, the master and the slave, and so on'. Instead, Foucault argues (1980, p. 198), 'power (in the substantive sense), l'pouvoir, doesn't exist,' which means that 'power is not a substance. Neither is it a mysterious property whose origin must be delved into. Power is only a certain type of relation between individuals' (Foucault 2002, p. 324). As a consequence, power cannot be 'located at—or emanating from—a given point':

> Power's condition of possibility, or in any case the viewpoint which permits one to understand its exercise, even in its more "peripheral" effects, and which also makes it possible to use its mechanisms as a grid of intelligibility of the social order, must not be sought in the primary existence of a central point, in a unique source of sovereignty from which secondary and descendent forms would emanate; it is the moving substrate of force relations which, by virtue of their inequality, constantly engender states of power, but the latter are always local and unstable (Foucault 1978, p. 93).

That is, power cannot be in the possession of anybody, be it a dominant class, sovereign, state or a subject. Instead, Foucault argues (1978, p. 94), 'power is exercised from innumerable points, in the interplay of nonegalitarian and mobile relations'.

> Power relations are both intentional and nonsubjective. If in fact they are intelligible, this is not because they are the effect of another instance that "explains" them, but rather because they are imbued, through and through, with calculation: there is no power that is exercised without a series of aims and objectives. But this does not mean that it results from the choice or decision of an individual subject; let us not look for the headquarters that presides over it rationally; neither the caste which governs, nor the groups which control the state apparatus, nor those who make the most important economic decisions direct to the entire network of power that functions in a society (and makes it function); the rationality of power is characterized by tactics that are often quite explicit at the restricted level where they are inscribed (the local cynicism of power), tactics which, becoming connected to one another, attracting and propagating one another, but finding their base of support and their condition elsewhere, end by forming comprehensive systems: the logic is perfectly clear, the aims decipherable, and yet it is often the case that no one is there to have invented them, and few who can be said to have formulated them: an implicit characteristic of the great anonymous, almost unspoken strategies which coordinate the loquacious tactics whose "inventors" or decision-makers are often without hypocrisy (Foucault 1978, pp. 94–95).

Foucault is drawing from Nietzsche (2002) to conceive of power as a purely relational thing. Power in this sense is not a matter of particular agents, but that which is in-between: 'it is a way in which some act on others' (Foucault 2002, p. 340), which constitutes 'a network of relations' (Foucault 1979, p. 27). As a consequence, one should not ask what power is and where it comes from, but how power operates, 'how is it exercised' (Foucault 1988, p. 102): 'to approach the theme of power by an analysis of "how" is, therefore, to introduce several critical shifts in relation to the supposition of a fundamental power. It is to give oneself as the object of analysis power relations and not power itself' (Foucault 1979, p. 28). The exercise of power can be defined 'as a way in which certain actions may structure the field of other possible actions' (Foucault 2002, p. 343). Insofar as 'power exists only in action' (Foucault 1980, p. 89), 'it is not the `privilege,' acquired or preserved, of the dominant class, but the overall effect of its strategic positions' (Foucault 1979, p. 27). More specifically: 'one has to be nominalistic, no doubt: power is not an institution, and not a structure, neither is it a certain strength we are endowed with; it is the name one attributes to a complex strategic situation in a particular society' (Foucault 1978, p. 93). Following from this, Foucault explains (2000a, p. 291), is that when he speaks about power he in fact always means the 'relations of power' that 'go right down into the depths of society'. In this sense, 'power comes from below' (Foucault 1978, p. 94):

> that is, there is no binary and all-encompassing opposition between rulers and ruled at the root of power relation, and serving as a general matrix—no such duality extending from the top down and reacting on more and more limited groups to the very depths of the social body. One must suppose, rather, that the manifold relationships of force that take shape and come into play in the machinery of production, in families, limited groups and institutions, are the basis for wide-ranging effects of cleavage that run through the social body as a whole (Foucault 1978, p. 94).

Hence, the analysis of power cannot 'assume that the sovereignty of the state, the form of the law, or the overall unity of a domination are given at the outset; rather, these are only the terminal forms power takes' (Foucault 1978, p. 92). Foucault, thus, radically overturns the prevailing top-down, centralistic, substantial concepts of power to introduce an un-substantial, relational bottom-up understanding of power, which he also calls the 'micro-physics of power' or the 'capillary functioning of power' (Foucault 1979). By taking all the above insights into account, according to Foucault (1978, p. 92), power must be understood:

> as the multiplicity of force relations immanent in the sphere in which they operate and which constitute their own organization; as the process which, through ceaseless struggles and confrontations, transforms, strengthens, or reverses them; as the support which these force relations find in one another, thus forming a chain or a system, or on the contrary, the disjunctions and contradictions which isolate them form one another, and lastly, as the strategies in which they take effect, whose general design or institutional crystallization is embodied in the state apparatus, in the formulation of the law, in the various social hegemonies.

Another important characteristic of Foucault's understanding of power is that he refuses the prevailing negative hypothesis of power, which conceives it only in negative terms as exclusion, prohibition or repression possibly coming from some 'superstructural positions' (Foucault 1978, p. 94, 2002, p. 120). Here, again, Foucault owes a great deal to Nietzsche (1989) in the Genealogy of Morals where he reversed and overturned the priority of the subject over power common to the tradition of Western metaphysics. Namely, Nietzsche and Foucault consider relations of power not as the repressive effect of the human subject, but on the contrary as having a 'directly productive role, wherever they come into play' (Foucault 1978, p. 94):

> If power were never anything but repressive, if it never did anything but to say no, do you really think one would be brought to obey it? What makes power hold good, what makes it accepted, is simply the fact that it doesn't only weigh on us as a force that says no; it also traverses and produces things, it induces pleasure, forms knowledge, produces discourse. It needs to be considered as a productive network that runs through the whole social body, much more than as a negative instance whose function is repression (Foucault 2002, p. 120).

While the micro-physics of power "runs through the whole social body," its ultimate productive grip is the individual human body: 'power relations have an immediate hold upon it; they invest it, mark it, train it, torture it, force it to carry out tasks' (Foucault 1979, p. 28). In this sense, 'body is the surface of the inscription of events' (Foucault 2002, p. 375). Insofar as the effects of power are thusly directly inscribed into human subjects, they are 'manifested and sometimes extended by the position of those who are dominated' (Foucault 1979, p. 28). It follows from this, Foucault explains (2000a, p. 291), that when he speaks about power he means the 'relations of power' that 'go right down into the depths of society' (Foucault 1979, p. 28): 'to approach the theme of power by an analysis of "how" is, therefore, to introduce several critical shifts in relation to the supposition of a fundamental power. It is to make oneself the object of analysis of power relations and not power itself'.

The productive and microphysical nature of power led Foucault (2000a, p. 291) to the conclusion that relations of power are present in all types of human relationships: 'The omnipresence of power: not because it has the privilege of consolidating everything under its invincible unity, but because it is produced from one moment to the next, at every point, or rather in every relation from one point to another. Power is everywhere; not because it embraces everything, but because it comes from everywhere' (Foucault 1978, p. 93). Hence, he does not think that 'a society can exist without power relations' (Foucault 2000a, p. 298). However, for Foucault (2000a, p. 298), the fact that power relations cannot be abolished from human societies is not a reason for pessimism and apathy since, according to him, 'power relations are not something that is bad in itself, that we have to break free of':

> Power is not evil. Power is games of strategy. We all know that power is not evil! For example let us take sexual or amorous relationships: to wield power over the other in a sort of open-ended strategic game where the situation may be reversed is not evil; it's a part of love, of passion and sexual pleasure. And let us take for example, something that has often been rightly criticized—the pedagogical institution. I see nothing wrong in the practice of a person, who knowing more than others in a specific game of truth, tells those others what to do, teaches them, and transmits knowledge and techniques to them. The problem in such practices where power—which is not in itself a bad thing—must inevitably come into play is knowing how to avoid the kind of domination effects where a kid is subjected to the arbitrary and unnecessary authority of a teacher, or a student put under a thumb of a professor who abuses his authority.

Foucault, thus, overturns the common formula that power is inherently bad and, hence, has to be abolished by resistance that would finally lead us to freedom. Namely, according to Foucault (2002, p. 342), 'there is not a face-to-face confrontation of power and freedom as mutually exclusive facts (freedom disappearing everywhere power is exercised), but a much more complicated interplay'. That is, Foucault does not perceive resistance and freedom simply as antipodes of relations of power, but rather coexistent with the relations of power.

> In order for power relations to come into play, there must be at least a certain degree of freedom on both sides./.../This means that there is necessary the possibility of resistance because if there were no possibility of resistance (of violent resistance, flight, deception, strategies capable of reversing the situation), there would be no power relations at all. This being the general form, I refuse to reply to the question I am sometimes asked: "But if power is everywhere, there is no freedom." I answer that if there are relations of power in every social field, this is because there is freedom everywhere (Foucault 2000a, p. 292).

Alternatively, as Foucault (2002, p. 324) argues elsewhere, 'there is no power without potential refusal or revolt'. This implies that, to be able to speak of relations of power, we have to acknowledge that 'power relations are possible only insofar as the subjects are free' (Foucault 2000a, p. 292). By free subjects, Foucault (2002, p. 342) means 'individual or collective subjects who are faced with a field of possibilities in which several kinds of conduct, several ways of reacting and modes of behavior are available'. If the field of strategic possibilities is closed and there is no possible points of freedom, we can no longer speak of relations of power: 'Where the determining factors are exhaustive, there is no relationship of power: slavery is not a power relationship when a man is in chains, only when he has some possible mobility, even a chance of escape (in this case, it is a question of a physical relationship of constraint)' (Foucault 2002, p. 342).

Resistance and freedom are—similar to power—without substance, which means that they too are purely relational. More precisely, they are directly related to power: where there are power relations, there are also resistance and freedom, and yet, or rather consequently, resistance and freedom are never in a position of exteriority in relation to power (Foucault 1978, 2000a). In other words, insofar as relations of power are everywhere in society, resistance and freedom are everywhere too.

This coexistence of power and freedom only holds on one level of Foucault's analysis of the relation between power, freedom and resistance. Namely, Foucault conducts his analysis of the relation between power, freedom and resistance on two levels. On the first more general level, Foucault (1978, 2000a) perceives freedom and resistance as ontological conditions of relations of power in the sense of constituting a field of strategic possibilities. On the other hand, the second level corresponds to a concrete actualisation of these strategic possibilities in the form of 'a way of behaving within a more or less open field of possibilities' (Foucault 2002, p. 341). While the first level is about 'a field of possibilities in which several kinds of conduct, several ways of reacting and modes of behavior are available' (Foucault 2002, p. 342), the second level tells us about what kind of conduct, what behavior is actually exercised. That is, on the second level of analysis, Foucault understands power, freedom and resistance as concrete practices, technologies, mechanisms and strategies that are in continuous struggle. In this case, power corresponds to concrete relationships in which an individual or a group of individuals 'try to control the conduct of the other' (Foucault 2000a, p. 292), and resistance corresponds to practices of resistance/liberation, through which people 'try to avoid their conduct to be controlled' (Foucault 2000a, p. 299). In other words, if 'power is games of strategy' (Foucault 2000a, p. 298), then the first level corresponds to the rules of the game and the dispositions of the players that constitute the field of possible action (which is determined by the outcomes of the previous strategic games), and the second level, to the mode in which the game is actually played. Outcomes of the game, then, again represent a new field of strategic possibilities, new rules and dispositions of the game and so on. In an actual situation, the two levels are closely and dynamically interconnected: a field of strategic possibilities indeed structures the field of possible action; however, it is through actual behavior that the field of strategic possibilities is either maintained or transformed. Therefore, Foucault explains (2002, p. 341), the exercise of power is always both 'a "conduct of conducts"[8] (corresponding to the 2nd level, L.Z.) and a management of possibilities' (corresponding to the 1st level, L.Z.).

Before we move to the connection between power and truth, we have to add that when analyzing relations of power, Foucault (2002, p. 337) insists that it is necessary to distinguish them from 'relationships of communication that transmit information by means of a language, a system of signs, or any other symbolic medium'. He argues that 'no doubt, communicating is always a certain way of acting upon another person or persons; however, in spite of the fact that 'the production and circulation of elements of meaning can have as their objective or as their consequence certain results in the realm of power, the latter are not simply an aspect of the former' (Foucault 2002, p. 337). That is, Foucault (2002, p. 337) is convinced that 'whether or not they pass through systems of communication, power relations

[8] Foucault uses the word conduire, which, convenient for his argument in French, means both to 'lead' others [la conduire] and to behave or conduct oneself [se conduire].

have a specific nature'. In this sense, Foucault argues (2000a, p. 277), it is also 'not enough to say that the subject is constituted in a symbolic system. It is not just in the play of symbols that the subject is constituted. It is constituted in real practices—historically analyzable practices. There is a technology of the constitution of the self that cuts across symbolic systems while using them'. As a consequence, Foucault (2002, p. 116) refuses the 'analysis couched in terms of the symbolic field or the domain of signifying structures,' and instead proposes 'a recourse to analysis in terms of the genealogy of relations of force, strategic developments, and tactics': 'Here I believe one's point of reference should not be to the great model of language (*langue*) and signs, but, rather, to that of war and battle. The history that bears and determines us has the form of war rather than that of a language—relations of power, not relations of meaning' (Foucault 2002, p. 116).

Truth (and Power)

According to Foucault (2002, p. 132), '"truth" is to be understood as a system of ordered procedures for the production, regulation, distribution, circulation, and operation of statements' and discourses[9]. A game of truth, then, corresponds to 'a set of rules by which truth is produced' (Foucault 2000a, p. 297). More specifically, 'it is a set of procedures that lead to a certain result, which, on the basis of its principles and rules of procedure, may be considered valid or invalid, winning or losing' (Foucault 2000a, p. 297). In order to grasp the workings of these 'principles and rules of procedure,' and to therefore understand 'how truth games are set up and how are they related to power relations,' Foucault (2000a, p. 296) posed 'the problem of knowledge and power' (2000a, p. 290). He explains, however, that the problem of knowledge and power was not the fundamental problem for him, but 'an instrument that makes it possible to analyse the problem of the relationship between subject and truth' in what seemed to him 'the most precise way' (Foucault 2000a, p. 290).

Truth according to Foucault does not have an objective or metaphysical value and does not correspond to an objective reality. Rather, truth is an effect of power (relations). Here, Foucault is also drawing from Nietzsche (1968, num. 481), who argued,

> Against positivism, which halts at phenomena -"There are only facts"- I would say: No, facts is precisely what there is not, only interpretations. We cannot establish any fact "in itself": perhaps it is folly to want to do such a thing. "Everything is subjective," you say; but even this is interpretation. The "subject" is not something given, it is something added and invented and projected behind what there is. Finally, is it necessary to posit an interpreter

[9] Insofar as Foucault understands statements as basic units of discourse, truth also corresponds to a system of ordered procedures for the production, regulation, distribution, circulation, and operation of discourses (for more on Foucault's understanding of statements and discourse, see Archeology of Knowledge). In this sense, the concepts of discourse (defined by Foucault (1978, p. 100) as a locus where 'power and knowledge are joined together') and knowledge are subsumed by the later Foucault under the broader concept of truth understood as one of the three axes of experience.

> behind the interpretation? Even this is invention, hypothesis. Insofar as the word "knowledge" has any meaning, the world is knowable; but it is interpretable otherwise, it has no meaning behind it, but countless meanings.-"Perspectivism." It is our needs that interpret the world; our drives and their For and Against. Every drive is a kind of lust to rule; each one has its perspective that it would like to compel all the other drives to accept as a norm.

What in a certain historical moment in a certain society counts as truth always corresponds to a product of a certain cultural and historical constellation of power-knowledge relations, through which certain individuals or groups of individuals succeed in establishing their own particular interpretation of the world as objective truth: 'Truth isn't outside power or lacking in power: contrary to a myth whose history and functions would repay further study, truth isn't the reward of free spirits, the child of protracted solitude, nor the privilege of those who have succeeded in liberating themselves. Truth is a thing of this world: it is produced only by virtue of multiple forms of constraint' (Foucault 2002, p. 131). Following from this, Foucault argues (1988, p. 107), 'instead of trying to find out what truth, as opposed to error, is, it might be more interesting to take up the problem posed by Nietzsche'. That is, 'how is it that, in our societies, "the truth" has been given this value, thus placing us absolutely under its thrall'?

Each society or a group of people in a specific time period has its own 'regime of truth' that articulates and determines 'the types of discourse it accepts and makes function as true' and 'the mechanisms and instances that enable one to distinguish true and false statements; the means by which each is sanctioned; the techniques and procedures accorded value in the acquisition of truth; the status of those who are charged with saying what counts as true' (Foucault 2002, p. 131). Moreover, truth is not only 'linked in a circular relation with systems of power that produce and sustain it' (Foucault 2002, p. 132), but—what is of even greater significance—also 'induces regular effects of power' (Foucault 2002, p. 131). In this sense, 'truth is no doubt a form of power' (Foucault 1988, p. 107).

In general, there are two main modes in which power and truth connect to individuals, thusly interweaving all three of the axes of experience together to 'transform human beings into subjects' (Foucault 2002, p. 326).

Truth and power can connect to the individual through 'the technologies of government' (Foucault 2000a, p. 299), where 'to govern, in this sense, is to structure the possible field of action of others' (Foucault 2002, p. 341). The technologies of government range from 'the way institutions are governed' right down to 'the way one governs one's wife and children' (Foucault 2000a, p. 299) and include systems and practices of control, coercion, incarceration and other mechanisms, techniques and practices of control that operate in conjunction with a certain regime or game of truth. Through the multiplication and intensification of such mechanisms and techniques, a more 'docile body' (Foucault 1979) or a more 'passive subject' is produced (Foucault 2000a, p. 291). According to Foucault, the subject is passive when it is caught in an extremely immobile network of power relations that significantly limits the field of possible action.

If the relations of power become fixed in such a way that they 'allow an extremely limited margin of freedom,' Foucault argues (2000a, p. 292), we cannot talk about the relations of power anymore, but we need to introduce a new concept—domination: 'When an individual or social group succeeds in blocking a field of power relations, immobilizing them and preventing any reversibility of movement by economic, political, or military means, one is faced with what may be called a state of domination' (Foucault 2000a, p. 283). States of domination 'are often established and maintained' through the technologies of government through which—as we have seen above—at the same time passive subjects are produced. Technologies or techniques of government, therefore, correspond to a level of power 'between the games (and relations, LZ) of power and states of domination' and are used to block the field of power relations. Foucault (2000a, p. 299) further explains that, consequently, what 'people ordinarily call power' in his theory of power actually corresponds to domination. Here, we have to note, however, that even though he distinguishes between relations of power and (states of) domination, the latter does not constitute a separate domain for domination is nothing but a fixation, an immobilization of otherwise more fluid relations of power.

The more power relations 'remain blocked, frozen' (Foucault 2000a, p. 283, 292) in a certain field of strategic possibilities, the less room there is for the possible exercise of freedom and resistance and the more dangerous they can become. In other words, power relations become particularly dangerous when games of strategy are played in a way that leads to a sudden or gradual immobilization of the relations of power resulting in the field of strategic possibilities becoming too asymmetrical. For Foucault, the power relationships as such are not dangerous in themselves. What indeed is dangerous is the immobilization of power relationships that results in closing the field of strategic possibilities. Metaphorically speaking, domination occurs when the rules of the game and the dispositions of the players are set up in a way that does not allow some of the players to play the game without considerable limitations or sometimes even completely preventing them to play the game: 'I can well imagine societies,' Foucault explains (2000a, p. 300), 'in which the control of the conduct of others is so well regulated in advance that, in a sense, the game is already over'. In the case of incarceration, for example (which is quite an intensive state of domination), prisoners are only left with limited points of resistance such as mutiny, escape or hunger strike. A state of total domination would then be a situation in which an individual has absolutely no possibilities for freedom or resistance. An example of total domination is a straitjacket, which prevents the individual even from performing the ultimate act of resistance: voluntarily taking his own life. For Foucault, putting someone into a straitjacket is, thus, not a power relation, but a physical relation of constraint.

Cases of such extreme domination, however, are quite rare in human relationships. It is much more common that even in the case of domination, the field of strategic possibilities permits at least certain points for possible resistance, which implies 'that we always have possibilities, there are always possibilities of changing the situation. We cannot jump outside the situation, and there is no point where you are free from all power relations. But you can always change it. So what I've said does not mean that we are always trapped, but that we are always free—well, anyway, that there is always the possibility of changing' (Foucault 2000a, p. 167).

In this sense, power relations are always 'mobile, reversible and unstable' ..., 'they can be modified, they are not fixed once and for all' (Foucault 2000a, p. 292).

The relations of power that are concentrated in a more or less intense state of domination can be modified through practices of resistance or 'practices of liberation' (Foucault 2000a, p. 282). Insofar as every strategic situation is specific, it also demands 'specific answers that take account of the kind and precise form of domination in question' (Foucault 2000a, p. 293). Foucault (1978, p. 96) explains his conception of resistance in this long, dense and often-cited quote:

> there is a plurality of resistances, each of them a special case: resistances that are possible, necessary, improbable; others that are spontaneous, savage, solitary, concerted, rampant, or violent; still others that are quick to compromise, interested, or sacrificial; by definition, they can only exist in the strategic field of power relations. But this does not mean that they are only a reaction or rebound, forming with respect to the basic domination an underside that is in the end always passive, doomed to perpetual defeat. Resistances do not derive from a few heterogeneous principles; but neither are they a lure or a promise that is of necessity betrayed. They are the odd term in relations of power; they are inscribed in the latter as an irreducible opposite. Hence, they too are distributed in irregular fashion: the points, knots, or focuses of resistance are spread over time and space at varying densities, at times mobilizing groups or individuals in a definitive way, inflaming certain points of the body, certain moments in life, certain types of behavior. Are there no great radical ruptures, massive binary divisions, then? Occasionally, yes. But more often one is dealing with mobile and transitory points of resistance, producing cleavages in a society that shift about, fracturing unities and effecting regroupings, furrowing across individuals themselves, cutting them up and remolding them, marking off irreducible regions in them, in their bodies and minds. Just as the network of power relations ends by forming a dense web that passes through apparatuses and institutions, without being exactly localized in them, so too the swarm of points of resistance traverses social stratifications and individual unities. And it is doubtless the strategic codification of these points of resistance that makes a revolution possible, somewhat similar to the way in which the state relies on the institutional integration of power relationships.

Insofar as power has no substance/source/centre and, therefore, cannot be in the possession of anybody, and insofar as points of resistance are, thus, 'present everywhere in the power network,' there is also 'no single locus of great Refusal, no soul of revolt, source of all rebellions, or pure law of the revolutionary' (Foucault 1978, pp. 95–96). According to Foucault (1979, p. 28), the overthrow of these 'micro-powers' does not, then, obey the law of all or nothing; it is not acquired once and for all by a new control of the apparatuses, nor by a new functioning or a destruction of the institutions. Instead, practices of resistance and liberation are in a continuous dynamic 'struggle' (Foucault 2000a, p. 167) with technologies/techniques of government and control. The momentary outcomes of these strategic games keep determining and redefining the field of strategic possibilities and vice versa: it is the current field of strategic possibilities that determines the possible field of action. If technologies/techniques of government are more pronounced, then they maintain the current field of strategic possibilities or may even further immobilize it. On the other hand, when practices of resistance and liberation are actualized, they can start opening up and "defrosting" the field of strategic possibilities to enable more points of freedom in its network. The more points of freedom there are in the field of strategic possibilities, the less domination there is. In this sense, resistance and liberation do not correspond to the abolition of power, but to the opening up of the field of strategic possibilities. In other words, insofar as according to the Foucauldian perspective resistance and relations of power are coexistent with each other, practices of resistance and liberation can only result in the abolition of domination (which corresponds to an immobilisation of power relations) and not in the abolition of relations of power as such.

Active Subjects, Freedom and Relationship to the Self

Above, we have seen that in the case of a more or less intense state of domination, it is first necessary to engage in practices of resistance and liberation that can open up the asymmetrical field of strategic possibilities (see Foucault 2000a, p. 168, 282). Only when the field of strategic possibilities becomes more symmetrical can we talk about 'power relations understood as strategic games between liberties—in which some try to control the conduct of others, who in turn try to avoid allowing their conduct to be controlled or try to control the conduct of the others' (Foucault 2000a, p. 299). In such a situation, truth and power connect more intensively to the individual through the 'mode of relation between the individual and himself' (Foucault 2000, p. 200), and they cause the subject 'to constitute itself in an active fashion' (Foucault 2000a, p. 291). The connection of truth and power to the subject in this case can be twofold and correspond to Foucault's distinction between the acts and the moral code where 'the acts (*conduites*) are the real behavior of people in relation to the moral code imposed on them' (Foucault 2000a, p. 263). That is, truth and power can establish and define a particular moral code or, more generally, particular guidelines for behavior. The moral code, however, is not crucial for Foucault. Namely, his historical analysis has revealed to him that in spite of the fact that 'the codes in themselves didn't change a great deal' throughout the history of Western culture, there were notably different subjectivities produced (Foucault 2000a, p. 266). As a consequence, Foucault argues (2000a, p. 263), 'there is another side to the moral prescriptions, which most of the time is not isolated as such but is very important: the kind of relationship you ought to have with yourself, *rapport a soi*'. Foucault (2000a, p. 263) calls this side of moral prescriptions ethics, which according to him 'determines how the individual is supposed to constitute himself as a moral subject of his own actions'.

According to Foucault (2000, pp. 262–265), the relationship to oneself (ethics) has four aspects. The first aspect, called the ethical substance, answers the question, 'Which is the aspect or part of myself or my behavior that is concerned with moral conduct?' The second aspect, called the mode of subjectivation, is the way in which people are invited or incited to recognize their moral obligations. The third aspect of the relationship to oneself is the telos, which tells us to which kind of being we aspire to be when we behave in a moral way. The means by which we can change ourselves in order to become ethical subjects is what Foucault calls the self-forming activities or technologies (practices) of the self, which constitute the fourth aspect of the relationship to oneself.

According to Foucault (2000a, p. 87), self-forming activities are the most important part of the relationship to oneself and can be defined as 'the procedures, which no doubt exist in every civilization, offered or prescribed to individuals in order to determine their identity, maintain it, or transform it in terms of a certain number of ends, through relations of self-mastery or self-knowledge'. More specifically, Foucault (1999, p. 162) believes that in all societies, whatever they are, it is possible to find

> Techniques which permit individuals to effect, by their own means, a certain number of operations on their own bodies, on their own souls, on their own thoughts, on their own conduct, and this is a manner so as to transform themselves, modify themselves, and to attain a certain state of perfection, of happiness, of purity, of supernatural power, and so on. Let's call this kind of technique a technique or technology of the self.

He further explains that there can both be relationships between these four aspects and also 'a certain kind of independence' (Foucault 2000a, p. 265). For example, he describes that 'there is no complete and identical relation between the techniques and the telos. You can find the same techniques in different telos, but there are privileged relations, some privileged techniques related to each telos' (Foucault 2000a, p. 268). As a consequence, an analysis of any mode of relation to the self has to identify the specific connections/independence of its respective aspects. All four aspects of ethics are closely interconnected to the power-truth because the aspects of relation to the self 'are not something invented by the individual himself: they are models that he finds in his culture and are proposed, suggested, imposed upon him by his culture, his society, and his social group' (Foucault 2000, p. 291). Moreover, 'they are frequently linked to the techniques for the direction of others' (Foucault 2000a, p. 277) and can be 'taken over to a certain extent by religious, pedagogical, medical, or psychiatric institutions' (Foucault 2000, p. 282).

Above, we have seen that while for Foucault power relations are not something inherently bad, they certainly can be dangerous if they become fixed and immobilized in a state of domination. Based on his critical analysis of the relationship to the self and practices of the self, Foucault also refuses to understand freedom as something inherently good in itself. While for Foucault an open and fluid network of power relations, which enables numerous strategic games between liberties, is undoubtedly much less dangerous than a state of domination, that does not mean that it cannot be problematic. Insofar as Foucault does not simply perceive freedom as something good and unproblematic in itself, he has 'always been somewhat suspicious of the notion of liberation, because if it is not treated with precautions and within certain limits, one runs the risk of falling back on the idea that there exists a human nature or base that, as a consequence of certain historical, economic and social processes, has been concealed, alienated, or imprisoned in and by a mechanism of repression' (Foucault 2000a, p. 282). Foucault (2000a, p. 282) strongly doubts such "transcendental" notions of inherent freedom of the human essence and programs of liberation according to which all that is required is to break 'the repressive deadlocks and man will be reconciled with himself, rediscover his nature or regain contact with his origin, and reestablish a full and positive relationship with himself'. Foucault (2000a, p. 282) illustrates his argument with the example of struggles against colonization:

> When colonized people attempt to liberate themselves from their colonizers, this is indeed a practice of liberation in the strict sense. But we know very well, and moreover in this specific case, that this practice of liberation is not in itself sufficient to define the practices of freedom that will still be needed if this people, this society, and these individuals are to be able to define admissible and acceptable forms of existence or political society.

So, why is liberation, understood as opening up the field of strategic possibilities, not sufficient? Why can an open network of power relations that has multiple points of freedom and that enables the subject 'to constitute itself in an active fashion' still be dangerous?

In order to explain this, we have to return to the dual-level analysis of the relation between power, freedom and resistance. Namely, we have argued that while the first level is about the field of possibilities in which several kinds of conduct are available, the second level tells us about what kind of conduct and what behavior is actually exercised. Insofar as domination limits the kinds of conduct available, it is dangerous on both levels. Freedom, on the other hand, can be dangerous on the second level. That is, even when the field of strategic possibilities (i.e. the first level) is considerably open, potentially allowing various kinds of conduct (like in contemporary Western societies), it can still be dangerous because 'in a society like our own, games can be very numerous, and the desire to control the other is all the greater—as we see in family relationships, for example, or emotional or sexual relationships' (Foucault 2000a, p. 300). Metaphorically speaking, while domination is dangerous because the rules of the game and the dispositions of the players are set up in a way that does not allow some of the players to play the game without considerable limitations, freedom can be dangerous on the level where the game is actually played: 'the freer people are with respect to each other, the more they want to control each other's conduct. The more open the game, the more appealing and fascinating it becomes[10]' (Foucault 2000a, p. 300).

This means that liberation understood as the multiplication of points of freedom in the strategic field of power relations 'is not in itself sufficient to define the practices of freedom that will still be needed' if individuals 'are to be able to define

[10] In order to critically reflect on how the relations of power intersect with the relationship individual has with oneself Foucault (2000a, p. 225) introduces the concept of governmentality, which corresponds to an 'encounter between the technologies of domination of others and those of the self'. According to Foucault (2000a, p. 300) the concept of governmentality 'makes it possible to bring out the freedom of the subject and its relationship to others—which constitutes the very stuff [matiere]of ethics': 'I am saying that "governmentality" implies the relationship of the self to itself, and I intend this concept of governmentality to cover the whole range of practices that constitute, define, organize, and instrumentalize the strategies that individuals in their freedom can use in dealing with each other. Those who try to control, determine and limit the freedom of others are themselves free individuals who have at their disposal certain instruments they can use to govern others. Thus, the bases of all this is freedom, the relationship of the self to itself and the relationship to the other'.

admissible and acceptable forms of existence' (Foucault 2000a, p. 282). What is needed are practices of freedom that correspond to concrete behavior (i.e. the second level). This is the reason why Foucault (2000a, p. 283) emphasizes 'practices of freedom over practices of liberation; again the latter indeed have their place, but they do not seem to me to be capable by themselves of defining all the practical forms of freedom'. As a consequence, Foucault concludes (2000a, p. 283), 'liberation paves the way for new power relationships, which must be controlled by practices of freedom'.

Here, we must note that the two modes described above (active and passive constitution of the subject) should not be taken as ultimately separate, but rather as representing the two opposite ends of a dynamic continuum on which the degree of fluidity/mobility of power relations determines whether subjects are constituted in either a more passive or active way. And on this continuum, Foucault explains (2002, p. 331), there are three types of struggles: 'against forms of domination (ethnic, social, and religious); against forms of exploitation that separate individuals from what they produce; or against that which ties the individual to himself and submits him to others in this way (struggles against subjection [*assujettissement*], against forms of subjectivity and submission)'.

In sum, a key part of Foucault's notion of experience is the idea that our experience—in the everyday sense of the term—is determined by forms of truth, power and relation to the self that are historically singular. The experience is, therefore, 'not a simple confrontation between a perceiving subject and a world of objects' (O'Leary 2010, p. 180). Rather, O'Leary explains (2010, p. 180), 'the forms of the subjective experience are to a large degree made possible by elements in the surrounding culture and society'. Following from this is 'that there is not even any subject existing independently of these elements and preceding the experience itself' (O'Leary 2010, p. 180). The subject is, hence, 'not the ground of possibility of the experience; rather, the form of subjectivity emerges in response to the occurrence of a whole range of experiences[11]. And these experiences, with their concomitant forms of subjectivity, have their own historicity' (O'Leary 2010, p. 180).

In our view, the experience of happiness represents an important part of the range of experiences that were and still are connected to the constitution of the subjectivities in Western culture. As a consequence the second part of the book shall attempt an analysis of the experience of happiness in Western culture, which can be conducted using genealogical and archeological tools.

[11] From an individual viewpoint, this range of experience corresponds both to a kind of synchronic range of various kinds of experiences understood in the broader sense as an a priori experience that an individual can potentially experience (such as the experience of happiness, madness, sexuality etc.) and also to a kind of a diachronic range of aggregated individual's concrete past experiences of different kinds.

Part II
The Birth of Happiness

Chapter 4
Middle Ages: The Time Before Happiness

Methodology: Genealogical Approach and Archeological Method

The archeological method was extensively developed by Foucault in Archeology of Knowledge (2004) and was his most preferred tool, especially in the 1960s. In the 1970s, due to his interest in Nietzsche and a shift of focus to the workings of power, Foucault started developing a new genealogical approach. Even though the relationship between archeology and genealogy was somewhat vague in Foucault's work in the 1970s, he always perceived genealogy as a broader concept. Eventually, it became quite clear that for Foucault, the genealogical approach subsumed archeology in the sense that it represents its methodological framework.

As we have seen above, the general theme of Foucault's research was the history of thought (understood in a wide sense). According to Foucault (1983), there is no other way we can have access to thought, 'either to our own present thought, or our contemporaries' thought, or of course thought of people of previous periods, but through discourses'. In this sense, Foucault (1983) uses archeology as a method to research a 'set of discourses, which has to be analyzed as an event or as a set of events'. Genealogy, on the other hand, Foucault explains (1983), 'is both the reason and the target of the analysis of discourses as events, and what I try to show is how those discursive events have determined in a certain way what constitutes our present and what constitutes ourselves: our knowledge, our practices, our type of rationality, our relationship to ourselves and to the others (Foucault 1983). As a consequence, Foucault concludes (1983), 'Genealogy is the aim of the analysis and the archaeology is the material and methodological framework'.

In order to better understand the specifics of Foucault's genealogical approach, we have to explore how he adopted and developed Nietzsche's understanding of genealogy. According to Foucault, Nietzsche's genealogical approach challenges the pursuit of the origin [*Ursprung*] and its metaphysics common to the historical approach in the traditional sense that we have described above. Nietzsche and Foucault (2000b, p. 371) are against the 'search for origins' because

L. Zevnik, *Critical Perspectives in Happiness Research*,
DOI 10.1007/978-3-319-04403-3_4, © Springer International Publishing Switzerland 2014

> it is an attempt to capture the exact essence of things, their purest possibilities, and their carefully protected identities; because this search assumes the existence of immobile forms that precede the external world of accident and succession. This search is directed to "that which is already there," the "very same" of an image of a primordial truth fully adequate to its nature, and it necessitates the removal of every mask to ultimately disclose an original identity (Foucault 200b, p. 371).

Genealogy that refuses to extend such 'faith in metaphysics,' on the other hand, discovers that there is no 'timeless and essential secret' behind things, but 'the secret that they have no essence, or that their essence was fabricated in a piecemeal fashion from alien forms' (Foucault 2000b, p. 371). Foucault and Nietzsche, therefore, propose an approach that could be seen as a kind of anti-essentialist or anti-positivist history. 'Genealogies,' Foucault argues (1980, p. 83), are 'not positivistic returns to a more careful or exact form of science. They are precisely anti-sciences'.

In this sense, genealogy also refuses another 'postulate of the origin'—that of 'the site of truth':

> The very question of truth, the right it appropriates to refute error and oppose itself to appearance, the manner in which it was initially made available to the wise, then was withdrawn by man of piety to an unattainable world where it was given the double role of consolation and imperative, finally rejected as a useless notion, superfluous and contradicted on all sides—does this not form a history, the history of an error we call truth? (Foucault 2000b, p. 372)

Rather than origin [*Ursprung*], Foucault argues (2000b, p. 373), descent [*Herkunft*] and emergence—the moment of arising [*Entstehung*]—are 'more exact' in 'recording the true object of genealogy'. According to Foucault (2000b, p. 374), 'the analysis of descent permits the dissociation of the Me, its recognition and displacement as an empty synthesis': 'where the soul pretends unification or the Me fabricates a coherent identity, the genealogist sets out to study the beginning—numberless beginnings, whose faint traces and hints of color are readily seen by a historical eye'. In this sense, Foucault explains (2000b, p. 374),

> Genealogy does not pretend to go back in time to restore an unbroken continuity that operates beyond dispersion of oblivion; its task is not to demonstrate that the past actively exists in the present, that it continues to secretly animate the present, having imposed a predetermined form on all its vicissitudes. Genealogy does not resemble the evolution of a species and does not map the destiny of a people. On the contrary, to follow the complex course of descent is to maintain passing events in their proper dispersion; it is to identify the accidents, the minute deviations—or conversely, the complete reversals—the errors, the false appraisals, and the faulty calculations that give birth to those things which continue to exist and have value for us.

As for emergence, Foucault continues (2000b, p. 376), we have to acknowledge that it 'is always produced in a particular state of forces'. While 'in placing present needs at the origin, the metaphysician would convince us of an obscure purpose that seeks its realization at the moment it arises,' genealogy, on the other hand, Foucault argues (2000b, p. 376), 'seeks to reestablish the various systems of subjection: not the anticipatory power of meaning, but the hazardous play of dominations'.

Contrary to the metaphysics of the traditional historical approach, Foucault (2000b, p. 379) adopts a historical sense, which 'evades metaphysics' and 'refuses the certainty of absolutes' that can produce what Nietzsche calls *wirkliche Historie*—"effective history". Given this, the genealogical sense of history 'corresponds to the acuity of a glance that distinguishes, separates, and disperses; that is, capable of liberating divergence and marginal elements—the kind of dissociating view that is capable of decomposing itself, capable of shattering the unity of man's being through which it was thought that he could extend his sovereignty to the events of his past' (Foucault 2000b, p. 379).

As such, the genealogical approach enables us to analyze history without assuming a priori foundations, essences, historical origins or absolute historical truths. In this sense, Foucault is close to Rorty's (1979) position of anti-foundationalism, but he also extends it to the historical perspective. Insofar as the Foucauldian genealogical approach (in a way similar to the postmodern anthropology) refuses the modern epistemology and the scientific approach, it doesn't claim to be producing objective knowledge about the world and history, but serious true fictions about history: 'Of course, there is no question of it being anything else but fiction,' Foucault (2002, p. 242) once commented on his work.

There are, however, some notable differences between the Foucauldian and anthropological fictions. The first is that while the "other" in anthropological fictions primarily corresponds to "other cultures," in Foucauldian fictions the "other" usually corresponds to our own (Western) culture in other (past) times. What is even more important is the difference in the purposes of fictions. While anthropological fictions are primarily of explanatory nature, Foucauldian fictions are explicitly conveyed to enable what Foucault calls a 'limit-experience,' which has the potential to transform the experience of its author and his readers.

'The distinctive feature of Foucault's histories, the feature which gives them their transformative power,' O'Leary explains (2008, p. 14), 'is the fact that they are not only descriptions of the past, but attempts to modify the present through a transformation, or a fictioning, of experience'. In this sense, Foucault explains (1990, p. 9), his 'studies in "history," are 'not the work of a historian,' but a critical 'philosophical exercise': 'The object was to learn to what extent the effort to think one's own history can free thought from what it silently thinks, and so enable it to think differently' (Foucault 1990, p. 9).

In order to better explain the Foucauldian genealogical approach and its fictions (in the spirit of which we are going to conduct our historical analysis of happiness in Western culture), we have to understand Foucault's specific relationship towards truth, which is based on his original critique of the modern relationship towards truth. While Foucault, in a similar way to Rorty (see Chap. 2), considers Descartes's philosophy as an important turning point in the history of Western thought that enabled the institutionalization of modern science and epistemology, he takes his critical reflection another step further.

The Critique of the Modern Relationship to Truth

In the course of his late theoretical development, Foucault's interest in antiquity shifted from the genealogical analysis of sexuality as a 'historically singular form of experience' (Foucault 1990) to a broader analysis of the historically different forms of experience of the relationship between the subject and truth (Foucault 2005). In order to reflect on modes of subjectivity and modes of relationship to the truth in Western culture, in his Hermeneutics of the Subject course at College de France, Foucault conducted a genealogy of the Western forms of experience of the relationship between the subject and truth. His critical undertaking can help us understand the historical currents that have determined the scientific relationship to the truth, which, according to Foucault (2000, p. 279), made 'possible the institutionalization of modern science' and at the same time lost the potential to 'save the subject' (Foucault 2005, p. 19). As a consequence, Foucault articulated an alternative critical mode of relationship towards truth, which is essential for the understanding of his genealogical approach and his historical fictions that are produced by it.

Before we can describe Foucault's relationship with truth, we first have to understand Foucault's analysis of the philosophical principles of care for the self [*epimeleisthai heautou]* and know yourself [*gnothi seauton*].

Foucault (2000a, 2005) notes that, in antiquity, modes of subjectivity were mostly not rooted in any firm formal external religious, ethical or legal rules; instead, the individual's behavior was regulated by an internal ethical relationship with oneself. Ethical reflection starts in antiquity exactly at the point where the rules, regulations and formal restrictions end. The relation with the self ('rapport a soi') was a matter of personal 'aesthetic' and/or 'political choice' (Foucault 2000a, p. 266). If one wanted to occupy an important position in society, to rule others or to live a good and happy life and leave an exalted reputation behind him, one first had to fashion oneself to give one's subjectivity a particular form. This was done through what the Greeks called 'epimeleia heautou' (care of the self).

Foucault (2000a, p. 256) did not uncritically consider antiquity a lost paradise and, hence, did not see it as an alternative because, according to him, 'you can't find the solution of a problem in the solution of another problem raised at another moment by another people'. Nevertheless, he was convinced that we could draw some useful inspirations and insights from it to solve our current problems.

Since we are analyzing happiness, it is especially the historical period of the first and second centuries A.D., which Foucault (2005) referred to as 'a golden age in the history of care of the self,' that is particularly interesting for our discussion. First, because in this period (like during most of antiquity) people were, as we are today, concerned with how to articulate the relation with themselves and others without founding it on a static religious or legal system and, second, because the care of the self at that time was 'a notion, practice and institution' whose objective was 'to arrive at happiness' (Foucault, 2005, p. 88). For people in this period, happiness and well-being were not matters of external factors (like the passive consumption of wealth, for example), but more a matter of actively cultivating 'a certain kind of constant relationship to the self, whether a relationship of mastery and sovereignty (being master of the self), or a relationship of sensations (having pleasure in oneself, experiencing delight in oneself, being content with oneself, etc …)' (Foucault, 2005, p. 86). As an outcome, care of the self 'involved arriving at the formation of a full, perfect, complete, and self-sufficient relationship with oneself, capable of producing the self-transfiguration that is the happiness one takes in oneself' (Foucault, 2005, p. 320).

Foucault explains that this care of the self 'does not mean simply being interested in oneself, nor does it mean having a certain tendency to self-attachment or self-fascination. The care of the self is a very powerful word, which means working on, or being concerned with something' (Foucault 2000, p. 269). The etymology of the expression *epimeleisthai heautou* (to take care of oneself, to be concerned with oneself, to care of the self) 'refers to a series of words like meletan, melete, meletai,' which mean 'to practice and train' (Foucault, 2005, p. 84). Specifically, 'epimeleisthai refers to a form of vigilant, continuous, applied, regular, et cetera, activity much more than to a mental attitude' (Foucault 2005, p. 84). This is because 'no personal skill can be acquired without exercise; neither can one learn the art of living, the *tekhne tou biou*, without an askesis that must be taken as training of oneself by oneself' (Foucault 2000a, p. 273). Moreover, if one wanted to be content with one's life, such activity of training should be practiced 'for the whole of one's life' (Foucault 2005, p. 87) starting early when still young and not finishing until one breathes his last gasp. To justify his argument, Foucault (2005, 87) cites Epicures: 'Who says that it is not yet time or that there is no longer time to practice philosophy, is like someone who says that it is not yet time or that there is no longer time for happiness'.

For Foucault (2005), the mode of the relationship between the principle of *epimeleia heautou* and the principle of *gnothi seaton* in different time periods is crucial for a genealogical illumination of our present relationship with the truth on which modern science is founded. Discovering the importance of *epimelea heautou* in antiquity, Foucault refutes the dominant readings of the history of philosophy, which hold that the Delphic prescription 'of gnothi seauton (know yourself) is undoubtedly the founding question of the relations between the subject and truth' in the history of Western thought (Foucault 2005, p. 3). Foucault (2005, p. 462) argues that, within the antique relationship with truth, gnothi seaton was subordinated to epimelea heautou, which in fact was 'the real support of the imperative know yourself,' because knowing yourself alone was not enough to access the truth: 'care of the self, precisely, is not just a knowledge (connaissance)' (Foucault 2005, p. 461). In order to be able to access the truth, a higher price had to be paid: 'for the subject to have right of access to the truth, he must be changed, transformed, shifted, and become, to some extent and up to a certain point, other than himself. The truth is only given to the subject at a price that brings the subject's being into play' (Foucault, 2005, p. 15). An evident conclusion of this type of analysis for Foucault (2005, p. 15) was the need to distinguish between philosophy and spirituality, which, in Western culture up to the sixteenth century, was 'always more or less obscurely linked' (Foucault 2000a, p. 279):

> We will call, if you like, "philosophy" the form of thought that asks, not of course what is true and what is false, but what determines that there is and can be truth and falsehood and whether or not we can separate the true and the false. We will call philosophy the form of thought that asks what it is that enables the subject to have access to the truth and which attempts to determine the conditions and limits of the subject's access to the truth. If we call this philosophy, than I think we could call "spirituality" the search, practice, and experience through which the subject carries out the necessary transformations on himself in order to have access to the truth. We will call spirituality, then, the set of these researches, practices, and experiences, which may be purifications, ascetic exercises, renunciations, conversions of looking, modifications of existence, etc., which are, not for knowledge, but for the subject, for the subject's very being, the price to be paid for access to the truth (Foucault 2005, p. 15).

For Foucault (2005), the transformative potential of truth for the subject in Western culture was lost when the centrality of care of the self was discredited and overshadowed by the principle of knowing yourself. He calls this event in thought the 'Cartesian moment' (Foucault 2005, p. 14), which 'disqualifies the care of the self and requalifies the gnothi seauton, dissociating a philosophy of knowledge from a spirituality of the transformation of the subject's very being by his work on himself' (Davidson 2005, p. xxiv). According to Foucault (2000, p. 279), by saying 'to accede to truth, it suffices that I be any subject that can see what is evident,' Descartes succeeds 'in substituting a subject as founder of practices of knowledge for a subject constituted through practices of the self'. Evidence is substituted for ascesis at the point where the relationship to the self intersects the relationship to others and the world'. Foucault (2005, p. 17) explains further,

> … we can say that we enter the modern age (I mean, the history of truth enters its modern period) when it is assumed that what gives access to the truth, the condition for the subjects' access to the truth, is knowledge (connaissance) and knowledge alone … I think the modern age of the history of truth begins when knowledge itself and knowledge alone gives access to the truth. That is to say, it is when the philosopher (or the scientist, or simply someone who seeks the truth) can recognize the truth and have access to it in himself and solely through his activity of knowing, without anything else being demanded of him and without him having to change or alter his being as subject.

According to Foucault (2005, p. 17), this does not mean 'that the truth is obtained without conditions.' Rather than 'spiritual exercises,' the modern science enabled by the Cartesian moment now requires two new orders of conditions defined only 'within knowledge' and 'neither of which fall under the conditions of spirituality' (Foucault 2005, pp. 17–18). They 'are either intrinsic to knowledge' (like formal conditions, objective conditions and formal rules of method) or 'extrinsic to the act of knowledge' (like the need to operate within a certain scientific consensus), but 'they do not concern the subject in his being; they only concern the individual in his concrete existence, and not the structure of the subject as such' (Foucault 2005, p. 18). Foucault believes that since the seventeenth century, philosophy has been developing 'a figure of the subject who is intrinsically capable of truth' (Gros 2005, p. 522) and, thus, 'superimposes the functions of spirituality upon the ideal of a grounding for scientificy' (Foucault 2000, p. 294). It is no wonder, then, that more than a century before Foucault Nietzsche (as Foucault's "educator") (1873, sec. 8) wrote in his essay "Schopenhauer" as Educator this: 'The only method of criticizing a philosophy that is possible and proves anything at all—namely to see whether one can live by it—has never been taught at the universities; only the criticism of words, and again words, is taught there'.

A consequence of this transformed relationship to the truth on whose legacy modern science operates is 'that access to truth, whose sole condition is henceforth knowledge, will find reward and fulfillment in nothing else but the indefinite development of knowledge' (Foucault 2005, p. 18). Such a 'Cartesian type of knowledge' can hardly be 'defined as access to the truth, but is knowledge (connaissance) of a domain of objects (Foucault 2005, p. 191), which, according to Foucault (2005, p. 19), cannot 'save the subject':

> Knowledge will simply open out into the indefinite dimension of progress, the end of which is unknown and the advantage of which will only ever be realized in the course of history by the institutional accumulation of bodies of knowledge, or the psychological or social benefits to be had from having discovered the truth after having taken such pains to do so. As such, henceforth, the truth cannot save the subject. If we define spirituality as being the form of practices which postulate that, such as he is, the subject is not capable of the truth, but that, such as it is, the truth can transfigure and save the subject, then we can say that the modern age of the relations between the subject and truth begin when it is postulated that, such as he is, the subject is capable of truth, but that, such as it is, the truth cannot save the subject.

For as long as modern science remains limited to intellectual clarifications and knowledge production within such a modern relationship to the truth, it will fail to make proper transformations of the subject. Namely, Gros (2005, p. 523) explains, 'according to the modern mode of subjectivation, the constitution of the self as subject depends on an indefinite endeavor of self-knowledge, which strives only to reduce the gap between what I am truly and what I think my self to be'. In this sense 'what I do, the actions I perform, only have value insofar as they help me to know myself better' (Gros 2005, p. 523).

As opposed to the modern understanding, the use and science in antiquity was (in line with their mode of relationship to the truth) fundamentally different. Theoretical and scientific understanding was secondary to and guided by ethical and aesthetic concerns: 'The one who cared for himself had to choose among all the things that you can know through scientific knowledge only those kinds of things which were relative to him and important to life' (Foucault 2000a, pp. 269–270). Scientific knowledge was, unlike in modern science, a matter of building indefinitely an objective system of knowledge, but was valuable to them only as far as it enabled them to integrate and use it to change their individual experience: 'the logos must actualize the soundness of action rather than the perfection of knowledge' (Davidson 2005, p. 528). Inspired by the Greek relation to the truth, Foucault was convinced that we have to try to refuse our contemporary relation towards truth marked by the Cartesian turn and adopt an alternative one that will enable us 'to put the subject back into the historical domain of practices and processes in which he has been constantly transformed' (Foucault in Gros 2005, p. 525):

> I think there is here the possibility of writing a history of what we have done, which can be at the same time an analysis of what we are; a theoretical analysis that has a political

> meaning—I mean an analysis that has meaning for what we want to accept, refuse and change of ourselves, in our actuality. In short, it is a matter of starting out in search of a different critical philosophy that does not determine the conditions and limits of a knowledge of the object, but the conditions and undefined possibilities of the subject's transformation.

It is precisely within such a relationship towards truth that the Foucauldian genealogical approach and its fictions are situated: 'Foucault clearly does not conceive of the writing of history as the faithful recording of the past; for him, the past is not so much another country as another tool—a tool with which to intervene in the present for the sake of a future' (O'Leary 2002, p. 96). If we put this in Foucault's (1980, p. 83) own words, he is aiming to 'make use' of knowledge about our history 'tactically today'. The genealogical approach, therefore, implies that when looking to the past, Foucault (1988, p. 262) is not interested in the problems of the past as historians in the traditional sense, but in the problems of the present: 'I set out from a problem expressed in the terms current today and I try to work out its genealogy. Genealogy means that I begin my analysis from the question posed in the present'.

Following Nietzsche (1968), who holds that the development of humanity is a series of interpretations, for Foucault 'the legitimate task of the genealogist is not only to record this history, but to offer a new interpretation, which will disassociate and dissolve the coagulated truths of the past' (O'Leary 2002, p. 100). This possibility, then, can simultaneously open up a potentiality for the transformation of the present and the future.

In this sense, Foucault explains (2002, p. 242), 'My problem is not to satisfy professional historians; my problem is to construct myself, and to invite others to share an experience of what we are, not only our past, but also our present, an experience of our modernity in such a way that we might come out of it transformed'. As a consequence, Foucauldian genealogies aim to produce fictions in the form of 'experience books' (Foucault 2002, p. 246). An experience book is

> 'a book that functions as an experience, for its writer and reader alike, much more than as an establishment of a historical truth'. For one to be able to have that experience through the book, what it says does need to be true in terms of academic, historically verifiable truth. It can't exactly be a novel. Yet, the essential thing is not in the series of those true or historically verifiable findings, but, rather, in the experience that the book makes possible (Foucault 2002, p. 243).

For Foucault (2002, p. 243), 'this experience is neither true nor false. An experience is always a fiction: it's something that one fabricates oneself, that doesn't exist before and will exist afterward'. Fiction, therefore, is not 'defined in opposition to truth' because 'it is possible for fiction to induce effects of truth, just as it is possible for a discourse of truth to fabricate, or to fiction something' (O'Leary 2008, p. 18). In this sense, O'Leary further explains (2008, p. 18), we must think of fiction 'in the same way we think of *poesis*; that is, as a fundamentally productive engagement in the world. To fiction is to fabricate, to produce, to bring into existence'. In his books, Foucault (2002, p. 244), thus, plays a 'game of truth and fiction,' in which 'the experience that the book makes possible is founded on the truth of its findings, but the experience itself is a new creation which may even, up to a certain point, destroy the truth on which it is based' (O'Leary 2008, p. 19).

According to Foucault (2002, p. 244), operating within a different relationship towards truth that favors concrete transformative effects for the subject over the quest for objective truth brings the following specifics to his approach: 'the first is that I don't depend on a continuous and systematic body of background data,' and the second 'is that I haven't written a single book that was not inspired, at least in part, by a direct personal experience'. However, Foucault continues (2002, p. 244), this 'is not at all a matter of transporting personal experiences into knowledge. In the book, the relationship with the experience should make possible a transformation, a metamorphosis, that is not just mine but can have certain value, a certain accessibility for others, so that the experience is available for others to have'. And last but not least: 'this experience must be capable of being linked in some measure to a collective practice, to a way of thinking' (Foucault 2002, p. 244). Following from this, the Foucauldian historical approach 'must be judged not only in terms of historiographical accuracy, but also in terms of the contribution it makes to the re-interpretation and re-constitution of ethical subjectivities today' (O'Leary 2002, p. 100).

The Foucauldian Understanding of Experience of Happiness

Inspired by Foucauldian theory, in this chapter we have articulated our own critical genealogical approach for the study of happiness that can significantly complement the existent approaches to the study of happiness in relation to culture, history and relations of power. In the following second part of the book, we shall make use of this approach to analyze the experience of happiness in Western culture.

If happiness is not a universal but culturally and historically specific experience, which is closely tied to the relations of power in society, then it follows that in order to understand happiness, one has to illuminate the historical process of its constitution/construction. Based on the Foucauldian understanding of experience and using his genealogical approach, we shall consequently analyze happiness as a culturally and historically specific mode of experience in Western culture. Here, it is crucial to emphasize that in contrast to the existent approaches to the study of happiness that perceive happiness only in terms of private internal experience (see, for example, Diener et al. 1997), the Foucauldian perspective enables us to examine happiness as an experience in a much broader sense. As O'Leary (2010, p. 163) explains, 'Foucault wishes to acknowledge and investigate the ways in which our experience exceeds our own private interactions with the world'. That is, the Foucauldian approach is not only interested in our private internal experience, but also in the shared 'historical a priori[1] of a possible experience for a period of time, an area and for given individuals[2]' (Foucault 2000b, p. 460).

---

[1] Here, we have to note that Foucault is not seeking the Kantian a priori, but the historical a priori and not all possible experience, but historically singular experience.

[2] Above we have seen that in addition to the wider understanding of experience as a shared a priori, the Foucauldian approach also implies the understanding of experience in terms of 'the ability to both account for and facilitate the transformation of experience through deliberate intervention'

The notion of a shared a priori of experience enables us to understand that our internal private experience is always 'made possible by larger social, political, and ethical (and, of course, cultural L.Z.) structures, which have their own historicity'. In other words, 'Foucault wants to bring together particular, everyday lived experiences with the larger epistemic, political, and ethical structures that make them possible' (O'Leary 2010, p. 173). In this sense, the Foucauldian understanding of experience points 'to the general background forms and structures that, in a general sense, determine, or at least set, the parameters for the everyday experience of people who live in a given period. So, it includes both these forms themselves and the range of actual experiences that individuals may have' (O'Leary 2010, p. 165). We shall, therefore, analyze the experience of happiness in wider terms as a general background and structures, i.e. a shared a priori of experience that sets the basic parameters for the everyday experience of happiness in Western culture.

Since we agree with Foucault (2005, p. 9) that 'the challenge for any history of thought is precisely that of grasping when a cultural phenomenon of a determinate scale actually constitutes within the history of thought a decisive moment that is still significant for our modern mode of being subjects,' our genealogical analysis in part 2 shall primarily focus on the historical processes that resulted in the birth of happiness in the seventeenth and eighteenth centuries, which in our view represents such a decisive moment. Namely, it was with the birth of happiness in the seventeenth and eighteenth centuries that after hundreds of years of Christian emphasis on the afterlife, our culture again started to envision the ideal of human existence predominantly in the mundane earthly realm, which decisively directed and fueled the modernization processes that determine what we experience today. Since this birth of happiness also constitutes a basic structure for all the later forms of experience of happiness in Western culture, we believe that such an undertaking is relevant not only because it can support the argument of the historical and cultural construction/singularity of happiness, but also because it will represent a valuable point of departure for any further inquiries into manifestations of happiness in our culture. In order to better understand the process of the birth of happiness and its result, the early modern experience of happiness, we will first examine the experience that preceded it. The main reason for such a wide chronological focus is that the experience of happiness in Western culture was, to a large extent, constituted in relation to the antecedent Christian experience. As a consequence, our analysis will chronologically span from roughly around the fourth century to the end of the eighteenth century, and it will include all three axes of experience described above.

Before we proceed to the actual analysis, we have to note that unlike Foucault who had the conditions and capacities to perform his genealogies mainly by analysing vast amounts of primary historical sources, our reach in this regard is somewhat limited. As a consequence, our genealogy of happiness will also make use of a fair amount of secondary historical sources. While on account of this our analysis

(O'Leary 2010, p. 164). With our analysis we therefore also hope to produce what Foucault calls an experience book. A book, that could result in a certain transformation of our experience of happiness and perhaps also in the transformation of experience of happiness of our readers.

will certainly not be as original and profound as Foucault's own work, secondary historical sources—which are now significantly richer and more inclusive than in Foucault's times—will enable us to examine a much broader time span.

In the start of part two (Chap. 4), we will examine what we shall call the Christian problematization of salvation and the experience of sin, which—as we shall argue—cannot be simply equated with the experience of happiness that only emerged in the seventeenth and eighteenth centuries. Chapter 5 will focus on a transitional period in the context of which certain new problematizations emerged that will eventually start constituting the experience of happiness. Finally, in Chap. 6, we shall illuminate the (birth) of experience of happiness itself. Following the Foucauldian methodological framework developed in Chap. 3, analysis will be conducted in every chapter in the second part of the book along the three interconnected axes that, according to Foucault, constitute the experience of any object: the axis of truth, the axis of relationship to the self and the axis of power. Accordingly, every chapter in the second part will be composed of three main subsections, each corresponding to one respective axis of experience.

Chapter 5
The Origins of Happiness in Renaissance and Reformation

While the late medieval period (from the 14th to the 16th centuries)—the topic of this chapter—was still largely characterized by the Christian problematization of salvation and intensive struggles around it, this turbulent period is nevertheless very important for the origin of happiness because it started opening up certain new problematizations that will be later connected to the (birth of the) modern experience of happiness.

Truth About Salvation in the Late Middle Ages

As a result of various interconnected catalysts, an 'astonishing doctrinal diversity' on the axis of truth about sin and salvation began to take shape from the 14th century onwards (McGrath 2004, p. 15). One such catalyst was the crisis of authority within the Church that intensified after the Great Schism of 1378–1417 between rival papal claimants, which resulted in a somewhat less repressive regime of truth. Weakened from within, the Church and its ecclesiastical authorities failed to maintain 'the normal methods of validation of theological opinions' and—as a consequence—were unable to 'take decisive action against heterodox views as and when they arose (McGrath 2004, p. 16). Such opening up of the regime of truth was even more dynamic given that at the same time new educational movements and rising professional groups in the cities throughout Europe were in rapid development 'steadily eroding the advantage the clergy once enjoyed over the laity (McGrath 2004, p. 12). 'An additional threat to the authority of the church understood at both the political and theological levels,' McGrath explains (2004, p. 12), 'arose from the rapid expansion of printing,' which 'permitted the transmission of ideas from one locality to another with unprecedented ease, and posed a formidable challenge to those wishing to ensure conformity to existing ecclesiastical beliefs and practices'.

In addition to the crises of the Church authority, 'the doctrinal diversity so characteristic of the later medieval period' was also related to several other developments' (McGrath 2004, p. 18). Namely, McGrath writes (2004, p. 18), 'It is clear that a number of quite distinct theological schools emerged during the thirteenth and

L. Zevnik, *Critical Perspectives in Happiness Research*,
DOI 10.1007/978-3-319-04403-3_5,

early fourteenth centuries, with differing philosophical presuppositions and methods. These schools tended to be based upon, or associated with, specific religious orders'. The Dominicans, for example, 'followed the teachings of Thomas Aquinas, the Franciscans those of Bonaventure, and the Augustinians those of Giles of Rome or Gregory of Rimini'. In addition, McGrath argues (2004, p. 19), 'local universities' were also influential 'in molding distinctive intellectual identities'.

Following from all this, 'There was considerable disagreement on the nature of the sources of Christian theology, and their relative priority' (McGrath 2004, p. 18), which included 'the absence of general agreement concerning the status and method of interpretation of both Scripture and the writings of Augustine of Hippo'. On top of this, a 'considerable confusion' reigned 'concerning the specifics of the official teaching of the church, with the result that doctrinal diversity arose through uncertainty over whether a given opinion corresponded to the teaching of the church or not' (McGrath 2004, p. 18).

Out of such a rich and diverse theological and social context, two important currents emerged, which can be seen as representing important steps towards the modern experience of happiness: humanism and renaissance and the Reformation movement. In the following, we shall argue that these developments began to problematize (good) feeling on earth and the affirmation of everyday life that will later (in the 17th and 18th centuries) constitute the modern experience of happiness.

The rich development of scholarship in the growing mediaeval cities and universities and the increasing number of lay scholars in the 15th and 16th centuries produced a social and intellectual movement called the Renaissance. Given that the Renaissance is characterized by its revival of the interest in what the Romans called the 'studia humanities'—grammar, rhetoric, poetry, ethics and history—that intensified the interest in 'man,' it has long been perceived as in stark contrast to what was believed to be the dark Middle Ages[1]. According to recent studies of the medieval period, there are sound reasons to believe that the change occurred 'in subtle modulations and tones' (McMahon 2006, p. 142). It is, hence, not surprising that the Renaissance hadn't produced any radically new ideal visions of human existence. That is, Renaissance philosophers were mostly consonant with the established Christian doctrine that perfect bliss is not attainable in this life, but only in the life to come, when man's immortal soul would enjoy the 'perpetual vision, contemplation and fruition of God' (Kraye 2007, p. 317). Even when drawing heavily on 'ancient philosophical sources in order 'to establish a system of ethics, which was appropriate for laymen living in the secular world of the present life,' they 'never forgot that these laymen were Christians, whose immortal souls were destined for a far higher goal in the next life' (Kraye 2007, p. 319). In this sense, Renaissance philosophers openly accepted and further elaborated the two-fold Thomist formula of perfect and imperfect beatitude. Emphasizing the dignity of man (like Pico dela Mirandola in his famous *De Dignitate Hominis* (1496)), they reinforced the role of human agency in the process of salvation and the consequent mitigation of the tragic effects of

[1] This view has been promoted by the influential 19th century scholar of the Renaissance Jacob Burckhardt (see Burckhardt 1945).

original sin underway since the 9th century (see, for example, (Desiderius) Erasmus of Rotterdam and his *Praise of Folly* (2008) and *On Free Will* (1969)).

Even though the Renaissance didn't produce any radically new visions of salvation, it certainly increased and intensified the interest in man. As Trinkhaus (1965, p. 42) observes, Renaissance philosophers produced 'an extraordinary large number of treatises' on themes such as human beatitude, misery and the greatest good. For our analysis, the most important consequence of such intensification of the interest in man was the beginning of the problematization of the realm of feeling—which will later constitute a vital component of the modern experience of happiness.

Already in 1431, Lorenzo Valla was quite surprisingly associating purely sensual pleasure with heavenly bliss:

> With the others, individual parts of the body are given pleasure as the palate by food, the nostrils by the rose and the violet; but with this kind, the whole body is partner to the pleasure. In this kind of joy, also, that is felt by not one but many senses; let it be touched upon only most briefly here because it relates to formerly mentioned matters, like your banquets, dances, and games ... In the state of eternal felicity that kind of pleasure will be much richer and more plentiful (Valla 1977).

It is important to emphasize that these new conceptions of heaven did not imply that human life in this world can become more heavenly like Aquinas's idea of double beatitude but vice versa: the visions of heaven were becoming modeled more and more according to positive feeling experienced on earth, which testifies to the start of a problematization of (positive) feeling during the Renaissance period.

An intensification of the problematization of positive feeling in the present life can also be observed in Renaissance painting. Although smiles already existed in Western painting and sculpture 'since the advent of Christianity,' McMahon explains (2006, p. 156), 'they were used only sparingly to brighten the faces of those known to enjoy certain beatitude: the blessed Virgin, Adam and Eve before the Fall, the angels, and the saints'. In the 15th and 16th centuries, however, Renaissance artists began do extend depictions of smiles and positive feeling to secular subjects. Leonardo da Vinci's famous Mona Lisa is just one example amongst many.

Valla's (1977) image of heaven (later accompanied also by other similar Renaissance descriptions and depictions of the afterlife[2]) was, therefore, at least 'in part a reflection of the greater acceptance of pleasure in the here and now' (McMahon 2006, p. 163). These, however, were only marginal developments limited to certain individuals or groups of people. The nascent problematization of positive feeling was still almost completely overshadowed by the dominant problematization of salvation and the experience of sin. When, for example, 'the aesthetic and libertine tendencies stimulated by the Renaissance' erupted in England 'in the aesthetic court of Charles I and the bawdy court of Charles II,' they 'were fiercely denounced by moralists and preachers as ungodly examples of aristocratic debauchery' (Porter 1996, p. 3).

The beginning of problematization of human feeling was not only becoming evident through a certain affirmation of good feeling and pleasure, but also

[2] See also Celso Maffei's Pleasing Explanation of the Sensuous Pleasures of Paradise (1504).

through their antipode: melancholy. Melancholy derives from the Greek melan (black) + chole (bile) and was first described by Hippocrates in the 5th century BCE and later elaborated by Galen in the 2nd century. 'According to late Medieval and Renaissance commentators who continued to regard Hippocrates and Galen as authorities on such matters,' McMahon explains (2006, p. 159), 'melancholy was one of the four principal humors that governed human physiology and mood'. In the famous *Anatomy of Melancholy* (1621), Burton collected and synthesized virtually all accessible knowledge from ancient times to his own, resulting in the following definition:

> Melancholy, the subject of our present discourse, is either in disposition or in habit. In disposition, is that transitory Melancholy which goes and comes upon every small occasion of sorrow, need, sickness, trouble, fear, grief, passion, or perturbation of the mind, any manner of care, discontent, or thought, which causes anguish, dullness, heaviness and vexation of spirit, any ways opposite to pleasure, mirth, joy, delight, causing forwardness in us, or a dislike. In which equivocal and improper sense, we call him melancholy, that is dull, sad, sour, lumpish, ill-disposed, solitary, any way moved, or displeased. And from these melancholy dispositions no man living is free, no Stoick, none so wise, none so happy, none so patient, so generous, so godly, so divine, that can vindicate himself; so well-composed, but more or less, sometime or other, he feels the smart of it. Melancholy in this sense is the character of Mortality.... This Melancholy of which we are to treat, is a habit, a serious ailment, a settled humour, as Aurelianus and others call it, not errant, but fixed: and as it was long increasing, so, now being (pleasant or painful) grown to a habit, it will hardly be removed (Burton 1621).

Central to our argument is the fact that by extensively reanimating classical sources, Renaissance humanists started perceiving melancholy not only as a natural and inescapable consequence of (original) sin, but also as a condition that can be cured or at least amended by human intervention. Moreover, many authors (including Burton) saw melancholy as a widespread social problem[3]. While it is impossible to assess to what extent their diagnosis was correct, it is clear that 'the diagnostic significance of the disease expanded in the sixteenth century, not in terms of its intrinsic medical-theoretical content, but in the extent to which it was deemed useful in a range of intellectual and cultural contexts' (Gowland 2006, p. 16). In this sense, the problematization of melancholy as a disease and the problematization of 'widespread melancholy in the population at large' can be seen as reflecting 'a growth of interest in psychology, especially in the passions of the soul' and, consequently, also the intensification of problematization of the domain of human feeling (Gowland 2006, p. 17). It is certainly worth noting that this new problematization was mostly not directly linked to the soteriological issues of salvation and the afterlife, but more with the betterment of the present life in the mundane realm.

As we shall see, these developments were 'further shaped by the Protestant and Catholic reform movements, which ensured that this increased attentiveness to psychological health became confessionalised, politicised, and visible in the public domain' (Gowland 2006, p. 17).

[3] It is interesting that this Renaissance diagnosis of widespread melancholy resemble the diagnosis of widespread depression in contemporary western societies.

The Reformation Movement

While since Augustine and the Council of Carthage, which formally interdicted the Pelagian doctrine, Christian doctrine clearly refused the possibility of true salvation on earth, certain themes from the Pelagian polemic endured. In particular, we have already seen that the issue of free will and the question of the role of human agency in the process of salvation drove many central medieval theological discussions about salvation. Insofar as after the Pelagian polemic the issue of Christian (im)-perfection had mostly been resolved, the main polemic around the issue of human (and church) agency in the process of salvation was centered around the issue of justification. Namely, while all theologians agreed that with the coming of Christ, the door to 'salvation shut in the Garden of Eden, was potentially open once more,' Marshall explains (2009, p. 42), 'contention raged' over the questions about 'how individual Christians might actually proceed through that door, the role of the Church in preparing them to do so, and whether the door was open for all or just for a few'.

The whole situation was further complicated by the fact that the doctrinal diversity and uncertainty in relation to the official teaching of the Church in the late Middle Ages was 'particularly evident in relation to the doctrine of justification' (McGrath 2004, p. 27):

> Such was the confusion concerning what constituted the official teaching of the magisterium and what was merely theological opinion that an astonishing diversity of views on the justification of humanity before God were in circulation at the opening of the sixteenth century. Those within the via moderna espoused a theology of justification that approached, although cannot actually be said to constitute, Pelagianism, while their counterparts within the schola Augustiniana moderna developed strongly—occasionally ferociously—anti-Pelagian theologies of justification (mcgarth 2004, p. 27).

In sum, 'an astonishingly broad spectrum of theologies of justification existed in the later medieval period, encompassing practically every option that had not been specifically condemned as heretical by the Council of Carthage' (McGarth 2004, p. 27). And it was precisely the doctrinal issue of justification and 'the rules and mechanisms of salvation' related to it (Marshall 2009, p. 42) over which the Lutheran Reformation began in the early 16th century.

Above, we have seen that since the 9th century and even more so after Aquinas, the ecclesiastical authorities were clearly endorsing the idea and practice that Christians can contribute (at least to a certain extent) to their salvation by performing good works and sacral rituals and by living virtuous lives. We have also seen that closely associated with such a vision of justification was the hierarchy of the sacred[4] and the belief that earthly suffering has a privileged position in the gradual ascent up the ladder to salvation in heaven. As a consequence, the centuries after Aquinas (especially 15th and 16th) were characterized by 'intense piety' (Greyerz 2008, p. 27) or even—as one theory suggests—by 'widespread and morbid "salvation

[4] This encompassed both places (certain places were holier than others), objects, and people (and their vocations).

anxiety[5]" … manifested in an intense, hyperactive, performance of piety' (Marshall 2009, p. 43). In this context, many people were keenly preoccupied with salvation and Martin Luther, an Augustinian monk and a professor of theology at Wittenberg, was one of them.

'The central term, to which Luther's deep spiritual trials can be pinned down,' Wriedt explains (2003, p. 89), 'is the "justice of God" that Luther understood as an active pursuit: the just God pursues the lawbreaker with wrath and punishment. The tested monk becomes more and more tangled in a vicious circle of exaggerated fear of sin and of works of repentance, which become perceived of as futile'. Although –by his own account—Luther was 'blameless, performing tremendous ascetic feats of fasting, self-flagellation, prayer and penance, he could never set his mind at rest'; for 'how could we be certain, he wondered, that we had performed enough good works to merit salvation' (McMahon 2006, p. 167). From a young age, Luther had suffered 'what he called tristia (melancholy or excessive despair)' (McMahon 2006, p. 165). Full of personal despair, he was questioning himself whether 'salvation was at all possible' and if he 'had not already been forgotten by God's grace, being condemned for all eternity' (Wriedt 2003, p. 89). Finally, while ardently contemplating book 1, verse 17, of Paul's Letter to the Romans, Luther experienced a personal revelation very akin to that of Augustine:

> Meditating day and night on those words, I at last, by the mercy of God, paid attention to their context: "In it, the justice of God is revealed, as it is written: The just person lives by faith". I began to understand that in this verse the justice of God is that by which the just person lives by a gift of God, namely by faith. And this is the meaning: the justice of God is revealed by the Gospel, but it is a passive justice, i.e. That by which the merciful God justifies us by faith, as it is written: "The just person lives by faith." Suddenly I felt that I was born again and had entered into paradise itself through open gates (Luther 1545 in Mcmahon 2006, p. 168).

In his illumination (significantly inspired also by his fatherly friend and vicar general of the order, Johannes von Staupitz), Luther realized that the possibility of contributing to one's own salvation by ardent penitential practices and self-torture was a source of suffering rather than the prospect of improving human condition. 'In view of God's free and necessarily given gift of grace,' Wriedt observes (2003, p. 90), 'Luther's striving for perfection, for pure love to God, for justification and holiness, proves to be absolutely wrong, even blasphemous. It appeared that he had rejected the caring love of the merciful God in favor of overconfidence in his own power to find happiness, that is, to acquire eternal salvation'. It, thus, becomes quite clear why 'in retrospect Luther accused his monastic teachers and ecclesiastical theologians of the way they spoke of Christ exclusively as the judge to whom account had to be given and good works had to be shown. Christ was not shown to his advantage as a comforter, savior, and redeemer but as a tyrant' (Wriedt 2003, p. 89).

Like Augustine centuries before him, Luther was unable to find peace by his own efforts. It is hardly surprising, then, that he was also in agreement with Augustine on account of the tragic consequences of original sin. Humans, for Luther (and also

[5] We could perhaps link this anxiety to the widespread melancholy diagnosed by Burton.

other reformers), are inherently sinful creatures unable to liberate themselves by their own efforts, and true salvation can only be bestowed by God's mercy in the life to come. In his view of justification, he, thus, returned to Augustine's logic and refused any possibility that human beings could be justified before God through their own merits. According to Luther, Greyerz explains (2008, p. 27), 'The only thing that justified the believer was faith in the exclusive efficacy of divine grace' and 'the sole means to that end was the understanding of faith on the basis of the Bible'. In the center of Luther's theology, we, therefore,

> Have the absolute sovereignty and freedom of God—expressed in such terms as grace, mercy, and righteousness—and across from him humans who are caught in their sin, completely incapable of taking any saving action. Sin hereby takes the expression of humans' perpetual attempt to place themselves in God's position and the desire to create and fulfill their lives out of their own power and responsibility (Wriedt 2003, p. 92).

According to Luther, 'This human overconfidence becomes most manifest in relationships with authorities from outside the Bible such as Aristotle and a Scripture interpretation led astray by church traditions lacking true theological back-up' (Wriedt 2003, p. 92). Following from this, Luther argued, 'The entire church of his day had fallen into Pelagianism[6], and thus required doctrinal reformation as a matter of urgency' (McGrath 2004, p. 25), hence the famous Protestant return to scripture.

On the basis of his doctrinal reformation guided by the idea of justification by faith that was posed directly against the idea of treasury of merit[7] endorsed by the official Church[8], Luther, and later the whole Reformation movement, opposed the majority of existent devotional practices and any form of indulgence issued by the Church (which included obligatory confessional practices). Following Augustine, Luther also adopted the notion of predestination, which was later even further radicalized by Jean Calvin, the second central authority of the Reformation movement.

Another important consequence of the doctrine of justification by faith was, Beutel explains (2003, p. 11), that insofar as faith would 'set humans free from the compulsion for self-justification,' it would also 'render them free to serve their neighbors'. While before good works have served personal sanctification, now they should serve the common good, as this was the only right way to serve and glorify God. Everyone, Luther preached, 'must benefit and serve every other by means of his own work or office so that in this way many kinds of work may be done for the bodily and spiritual welfare of the community…' (Luther in Lindberg 2003, p. 170). This aspect was even more pronounced in the Calvinist idea of the calling according to which 'in addition to the general calling to be a believing Christian, everyone

---

[6] Here, it is worth mentioning that given the vast doctrinal diversity and the confusion, according to McGarth (2004, p. 25), 'It could be argued that Luther's comprehensive theological protest against the church of his day was the consequence of an improper identification of the theological opinions of the via concerning the justification of humanity before God (opinions which he came to regard as Pelagian) with the official teaching of the church'.

[7] The idea of treasury of merits was already described above in 9.2.1.

[8] We shall analyze the effects of this development for the constellation of power relations bellow in the section about power.

had a particular calling, the specific form of labour to which God summoned him or her' (Taylor 2001, p. 223). Compared to the Catholic concept of vocation that was mostly related to priesthood and monastic life and implied the "hierarchy of the sacred," the idea of the calling maintained that 'all callings were equal, whatever their place in the social hierarchy, as long as they were of benefit to fellow humans (Taylor 2001, p. 223).

Initially, the church reform triggered by Luther 'took hold in the urban areas—at first among humanists as the representatives of the comparatively small urban educated class' (von Greyerz 2008, p. 28). But, 'what made the reform of the church into a true Reformation, into a socioreligious mass movement,' von Greyerz explains (2008, p. 28), 'was the fact that clerics, as preachers, began to adopt the Wittenberg reformer's ideas, in some cases perhaps merely his call for resistance to the existing conditions within the church'[9]. Spreading with the help of print-like fire throughout Europe, the Reformation movement soon diversified into regional variations 'carried by local reformist currents that had deep roots in the urban artisanal class, and in which the zeal for religious reform not infrequently merged with anticlericalism and political resentment of the governing class of councilors' (von Greyerz 2008, p. 28).

According to Greyerz (2008, p. 30), after 1525, we already have to 'distinguish between the radical Reformation, which would become a catch-basin for Anabaptists, Spiritualists, and Antitrinitarians, and the "established" Reformation, with the latter divided once again into a Lutheran and a Zwinglian movement. The main two currents were joined in the 1540s by Calvinism, 'which radiated outward from Geneva, and which, needless to say, had much in common with Zwinglianism' (Greyerz 2008, p. 30). Given the diversity of reformed churches and doctrines, we shall not go into the details of each of them. Rather, we shall mostly focus on Lutheranism and Calvinism, which represent the two main reformed churches and examine their contribution towards the birth of the modern experience of happiness.

Trying to counter Pelagianism, which they attributed to the official Catholic Church and to neutralize salvation anxiety catalyzed by the Church through the idea of earning of merit, the Reformation theologians have—resembling Augustine's vigor in fighting the Pelagian doctrine—also swayed far to the other extreme. They emphasized the tragic consequences of the original sin due to which humanity has lost free will and has become totally dependent on the merciful attention of God:

> For if we believe it to be true, that God fore-knows and fore-ordains all things; that He can be neither deceived nor hindered in His Prescience and Predestination; and that nothing can take place but according to His Will, (which reason herself is compelled to confess;) then, even according to the testimony of reason herself, there can be no "Free-will"—in man,—in angel,—or in any creature (Luther 1969, sect. CLXVII).

In this sense, reformation was aimed directly against the prevailing current of gradual reinforcement of free will and human agency in the process of salvation under way since the 9th century, intensified by Aquinas and culminating in the

[9] As we shall see in the chapter about power, according to Foucault (2007), these existing conditions mostly correspond to the existing modality of pastoral power institutionalized in the Church.

Renaissance movement[10]. Insofar as this current can be seen as a slow erosion of the tragic consequences of original sin and consequently as a certain rehabilitation of the standing of life in this world (like Aquinas's double beatitude or renaissance problematization of positive feeling), reformation could hence be regarded as a regression in the possibilities to improve the human condition in the present life. A closer inspection, however, reveals that this was not the case. First, the radical position on free will only pertains to man's relation to the divine and salvation in the afterlife, but not to his dealings with worldly things. Second, rather than connecting it to fatalism, the Reformers saw the lack of free will more like a neutralization of the existent salvation anxiety or like a certain catharsis in knowing that salvation does not depend on free will:

> I frankly confess that, for myself, even if it could be, I should not want free-will to be given to me, nor anything to be left in my own hands to enable me to endeavor after salvation; not merely because in the face of so many dangers, and adversities, and assaults of devils, I could not stand my ground and hold fast my free-will (for one devil is stronger than all men, and on these terms no man could be saved); but because, even were there no dangers, adversities, or devils, I should still be forced to labor with no guarantee of success, and to beat my fists at the air. If I lived and worked to all eternity, my conscience would never reach comfortable certainty as to how much it must do to satisfy God. Whatever work I had done, there would still be a nagging doubt as to whether it pleases God, or whether He required something more. The experience of all who seek righteousness by works proves that; and I learned it well enough myself over a period of many years, to my own great hurt. But now that God has taken my salvation out of the control of my own will, and put it under the control of His, and promised to save me, not according to my working or running, but according to His own grace and mercy, I have the comfortable certainty that He is faithful and will not lie to me, and that He is also great and powerful, so that no devils or opposition can break Him or pluck me from Him (Luther 1969, sect. XVIII).

Following from this, the Protestant radical refusal of free will along with the doctrine of justification by faith has resulted in the Protestant affirmation of everyday life, which, in our view, represents the second major current (besides the current of reinforcement of free will) that has eventually resulted in the birth of the modern experience of happiness.

The Affirmation of Mundane Life

Above, we have seen that already in the 9th century, the Church elites feared that the complete refusal of human agency in the process of salvation would erode the role of the Church as the exclusive mediator between God and the people, thus fundamentally transforming the established outlook of pastoral power. The Protestant return to Augustine and their rejection of free will has proved that their fears indeed had been justified.

---

[10] The best example of this is a written polemic on free will between Erasmus of Rotterdam (probably one of the most famous Renaissance thinkers) and Luther (see Luther and Erasmus 1969).

Maintaining the notion of free will in relation to the idea of treasury of merits, medieval Catholicism managed to firmly establish the idea that 'the church is the locus and vehicle of the sacred' and that 'we are brought closer to God by the very fact of belonging and participating in its sacramental life' (Taylor 2001, p. 216). Grace can only 'come to us mediately through the church, and we can mediate grace to each other, as the lives of the saints enrich the common life on which we all draw' (Taylor 2001, p. 216).

Insofar as the Reformers claimed that grace cannot be earned, but is freely given by the merciful God, they have rejected such mediation and the sacramental life connected with it. In their view, 'each person stands alone in relation to God: his or her fate—salvation or damnation—is separately decided' (Taylor 2001, p. 216). Along with the sacramental life, then, 'went the whole notion of the sacred in mediaeval Catholicism, the notion that there are special places or times or actions where the power of God is more intensely present and can be approached by humans' (Taylor 2001, p. 216). Following from this, 'Protestant (particularly Calvinist) churches swept away pilgrimages, veneration of relics, visits to holy places, and a vast panorama of traditional Catholic rituals and pieties,' that in their view 'impeded direct confrontation with the divine' (McMahon 2006, p. 170). 'And along with the sacred,' Taylor argues (2001, p. 216), also 'went the mediaeval Catholic understanding of the church as the locus and vehicle of the sacred'.

This transformation was closely connected to the Protestant refusal of special ecclesial vocations, which had represented an important part of mediaeval Catholicism. The celibate life in particular had been seen 'as part of the economy of the sacred' (Taylor 2001, p. 217). Namely, 'the medieval Catholic church viewed the celibate life as a meritorious work for salvation, and perpetuated patristic suspicions of sexuality as the font of original sin' (Lindberg, 2003 p. 168). Taylor (2001, p. 217) believes 'this was partly because of the connection between priesthood and celibacy, and partly because of the role of religion in an economy of mutual mediation: monks and nuns prayed for everyone, just as the laity worked, fought, and governed for the whole'. It was, hence, commonly accepted that the ecclesial vocations 'supposed a hierarchy of nearness to the sacred, with the religious life being higher/closer than the secular,' the result of which 'was a lesser spiritual status for lay life, particularly that of productive labor and the family' (Taylor 2001, p. 217). On the basis of hierarchy of the sacred, Foucault argues (2007, p. 268), medieval Catholicism was characterized by the existence of 'two clearly distinguished categories of individuals, clergy and laity, who do not have the same civil rights, obligations, or privileges, of course, but who do not even have the same spiritual privileges'. [11]

By rejecting the sacred and the idea of ecclesial mediation, the Reformers also rejected this hierarchy; spiritual privileges of the clergy and mandatory clerical celibacy, which, understood in this sense, 'was not just a matter of breaking church

[11] Here, we should add that, according to Foucault (2007, p. 268), the hierarchy of the sacred and the consequent hierarchical distinction between the laity and the clerics was actually a result of the institutionalization of pastoral power. As such, it should also be seen as one of the central points and outcomes of pastoral struggles in the context of the Reformation movement.

law,' but also encompassed the new evangelical understanding of the relationship to God and the world' (Lindberg 2003, p. 168). As Taylor (2001, p. 221) explains, 'The crucial potentiality here was that of conceiving the hallowing of life not as something which takes place only at the limits, as it were, but as a change which can penetrate the full extent of mundane life'. In other words, 'The rejection of the sacred and of mediation together led to an enhanced status for (what had formerly been described as) profane life' (Taylor 2001, p. 216). And once this potentiality for the affirmation of everyday life was realized, Taylor observes (2001, p. 221),

> It took on a life of its own. Its influence, in other words, was felt beyond the boundaries of protestant europe and not necessarily most strongly within these boundaries. It was felt in catholic countries, and then later also in secularized variants. Its impact was the greater in that it dovetailed nicely with the anti-hierarchical side of the gospel message. The integral sanctification of ordinary life couldn't consist with the notion of hierarchy, at first of vocation and later even of social caste. The gospel notion that the orders of this world, the spiritual as much as the temporal, are reversed in the kingdom of god, that the foolishness of the children of god is stronger that the wisdom of the wise, had its effect in discrediting earlier notions of superiority and accrediting the new spiritual status of the everyday.

The Protestant affirmation of ordinary life and their emphasis on the service for the common good also went hand in hand with the emerging scientific revolution pioneered by Francis Bacon. The reasons for such an alliance were mostly related to the fact that both movements 'saw themselves as rebelling against a traditional authority which was merely feeding on its own errors and as returning to the neglected sources: the Scriptures on one hand, experimental reality on the other' (Taylor 2001, p. 230). As a consequence, they 'both appealed to what they saw as living experience against dead received doctrine—the experience of personal conversion and commitment, or that of direct observation of nature's workings' (Taylor 2001, p. 230). As Lowe (2002, p. 18) explains, 'Bacon, in his *Novum organum* (1620), had recommended that we discover Nature's secrets by interrogating her systematically—essentially, by applying an inductive method of discovery through controlled experiment and observation'.

Within the framework of (Puritan) Protestant movement, Baconian science and its 'instrumental stance towards the world' gains a pious purpose not only in the obvious way—that it contributes to the right service in our use of God's creation (that is, to the general welfare of mankind), but also 'to his greater glory, as we come to understand his purposes and can render him knowledgeable and fitting praise for the marvels of his design' (Taylor 2001, p. 232). Making such an instrumental stance towards the world central, Taylor explains, 'could not but transform the understanding of the cosmos from an order of signs or Forms, whose unity lies in their relation to a meaningful whole, into an order of things producing reciprocal effects in each other, whose unity in God's plan must be that of interlocking purposes'.

According to Taylor (2001, p. 14), 'this affirmation of ordinary life, although not uncontested and frequently appearing in secularized form, has become one of the most powerful ideas in modern civilization' and as such a constitutive part of what was later established as the modern experience of happiness. This connection becomes even more evident when we consider that the affirmation of everyday life is also closely associated with the Protestant problematization and affirmation of the mundane good feeling, with which we shall deal in the next chapter concerned with the late medieval relationship to the self. Based on somewhat different foundations than the Renaissance,[12] reformation, thus, also contributed to the reinforcement of the general trend towards the intensification of the problematization of feeling in the present life. Let us now turn to the analysis on the axis of ethics and examine the affirmation of everyday life and the problematization of good feeling in the context of the late medieval relationship to the self.

The Attack on the Privileged Position of Suffering

Based on the affirmation of everyday life, the Reformation didn't have much difficulty in joining the trend of the problematization of (good) feeling in the present life already initiated by the Renaissance. Realizing that striving for eternal salvation through one's own efforts is a source of suffering rather that a path to eternal bliss, Luther entirely surrenders to God's mercy. Following from this, he believes, is not only a theological illumination, but also an opening up of the possibility of a good feeling in the present life:

> Faith is a work of God in us which changes and brings us to birth anew from God [cf. John 1]. It kills the old Adam, makes us completely different people in heart, mind senses, and all our powers, and brings the holy spirit with it. What a living, creative, active, powerful thing is faith! … [It] is a living, unshakeable confidence in God's grace; it is so certain, that someone would die a thousand times for it. This kind of trust in and knowledge of God's grace makes a person joyful [frohlich], confident, and gay [lustig] with regard to God and all creatures. This is what the Holy Spirit does by faith (Luther 1545).

Arguing that salvation is received rather than achieved, Luther and other reformers, thus, also radically questioned the privileged position of suffering in the Christian tradition. While the reformers did not deny earthly suffering (after all, they believed in the tragic consequences of original sin), they didn't see it as a path to salvation either[13]. Insofar as salvation is God's free gift, and not something earned by human effort, suffering was no longer perceived as a path to salvation. As a consequence, 'Luther and Protestants more generally dismissed with contempt the heroic ascetic

---

[12] Of course, there are also certain connections between renaissance and reformation (see McGrath 2004).

[13] Following from this the reformed tradition appreciated the created order and did not directly condemn the realm of sensual pleasures: 'on the one hand, through cross-bearing we are crucified to the world and the world to us. On the other hand, devout Christians enjoy this present life, albeit with due restraint and moderation, for they are taught to use things in this world for the purpose that God intended them' (Beeke 2004, p. 143). The reformers therefore opted for the middle way and advised their followers to avoid two opposite extremes: 'they must spurn the monkish error of renouncing the things of this world' (Taylor 2001, p. 222) and at the same time be careful not to become too absorbed in things of this world.

embrace: no more hair shirts, no more fasting, no more ecstasies of pain' (Mcmahon 2006, p. 172).

In the world full of suffering, we poor sinners, rather, have to cherish all the joy we can find. While we cannot strive for our ultimate salvation in heaven, we indeed—in spite of our sinful nature—can to a certain extent hope for moments of personal joy in our earthly existence. In other words, it is precisely the abandoning of the pretentious effort to reach salvation that opens up the possibility to experience something that has hitherto been deemed a sin and an obstacle to salvation: joy and good feeling in the present life coming from our deep faith in the mercy of God. While before earthly suffering was understood as a means towards perfect bliss on earth, now the unconditional faith in God's mercy and the hope of the life to come gives purpose to and a certain degree of enjoyment in our present life. This aspect of the Protestant transformative message is most evident in Luther's letter to the young Prince Joachim von Anhalt suffering from melancholy and despair at a young age like he did:

> Serene Prince, gracious Lord! [A mutual friend] has told me that your Grace has been a little unwell, but are now, thank God, again in good condition. It often occurs to me that, as your Grace leads a quiet life, melancholy and sad thoughts may be the cause of such indisposition; wherefore I advise your Grace, as a young man, to be merry [frolich], to ride, hunt, and keep good company, who can cheer your Grace in a godly and honorable way. For loneliness and sadness are simple poison and death, especially in a young man … No one knows how it hurts a young man to avoid joy [Freude] and cultivate solitude and melancholy … Joy and good humor, in honor and seemliness, is the best medicine for a young man, yea for all man. I, who have hitherto spent my life in mourning and sadness, now seek and accept joy whenever I can find it. We now know, thank God, that we can be merry with a good conscience, and can use God's gifts with thankfulness, inasmuch as he has made them for us and is pleased to have us enjoy them. If I have not hit the cause of your Grace's indisposition and have thereby done you a wrong, your grace will kindly forgive my mistake. For truly I thought your Grace might be so foolish as to think it is a sin to be merry, as I have often done and still do at times … Your Grace should be joyful [frohlich] in all things, inwardly in Christ and outwardly in God's gifts; for he gives them to us that we may have pleasure in them and thank him for them (Luther 1534 in Mcmahon 2006, p. 165).

It is certainly true that for Luther (and also other reformers), perfect salvation is not achievable by our human efforts. However, we can see from his letter to the young prince that this does not hold for the earthly experience of joy and happiness (gluck), which according to Luther can or even should be pursued (by our own efforts) in this world. Calvin (2002, p. 503) preached in a very similar way to Luther: 'if the praise of the Lord and thanksgiving can emanate only from a cheerful and gladdened breasts and there is nothing which ought to interrupt these feelings in us, it is clear how necessary it is to temper the bitterness of the cross with spiritual joy'.

Compared to Aquinas's imperfect beatitude, the Protestant joy is, therefore, much more profane/mundane than the Catholic imperfect beatitude. In the Thomist gradualist perspective towards salvation, imperfect beatitude refers to the partial ascent up the ladder of being and in this sense—as the name suggests—to a kind of partial/imperfect salvation on earth directly connected to the perfect bliss in heaven. For Aquinas, achieving a certain level of heavenly purity and virtue already in earthly life makes the present life more heavenly and gradually brings us closer to heaven. 'In contrast to all pieties of achievement, then and now,' the reformers, on the other hand, 'affirmed God's descent in Jesus to us rather than our striving to ascend to God' (Lindberg 2003, p. 165). As a consequence, 'the fullness of Christian existence was to be found within the activities of this life, in one's calling and in marriage and the family' (Taylor 2001, p. 18). This also meant that the reformed tradition appreciated the created order and did not directly condemn the realm of sensual pleasures. As Beeke (2004, p. 143) explains, 'On the one hand, through cross-bearing, we are crucified to the world and the world to us. On the other hand, devout Christians enjoy this present life, albeit with due restraint and moderation, for they are taught to use things in this world for the purpose that God intended them'. The reformers, therefore, opted for the middle way and advised their followers to avoid two opposite extremes: 'they must spurn the monkish error of renouncing the things of this world' (Taylor 2001, p. 222) and, at the same time, be careful not to become too absorbed in things of this world[14].

In this sense, when referring to joy and happiness coming from our faith in God, the reformed tradition (Luther in particular) is mostly not using these terms in a direct connection to salvation in the afterlife, but is positioning them in the registry of mundane earthly experience. While true salvation and bliss are still seen as pertaining to the afterlife, personal relief from the anxiety of salvation opens up and affirms a positive mode of earthly experience, which comes from 'living unshakable confidence in God's grace' (Luther 1545).

Like the Renaissance, but along a completely different path, the Reformation movement, therefore, also contributed to the problematization of (good) human feeling in the present life. While in the case of the Renaissance, this development was mostly driven by an increased interest in man, the reengagement of ancient philosophers and the further affirmation of rationality and free will, the Reformation reinforced the problematization of human feeling mostly in relation to the doctrine of justification by faith and the consequent affirmation of mundane life.

While indeed the Reformation, in general, stopped regarding good feeling on earth as a sin (and refused the privileged status of suffering inherent in the Catholic tradition), we have to emphasize that good feeling on earth was still far from being attributed a major role in the ideal of human existence. In other words, even though reformation and its affirmation of everyday life (like the renaissance before it) to a certain extent began to affirm good human feeling in the present life, salvation

[14] In relation to sensual pleasures, it is possible to observe an interesting, somewhat paradoxical difference between the Catholic and the Protestant tradition. In the Catholic tradition (in theory at least), the desire for the sensual has to be completely neutralized. Given that this imperative is obviously impossible to put into practice, there is always a certain leeway for occasional (either individual or collective) transgression (like medieval carnivals). While the idea of Vice and various penitential practices in this sense serve as an absolution for such transgressions, in turn, the possibility of an absolution also opens up a wider space for occasional sensual transgressions. On the other hand, the Protestant tradition in theory does not entirely condemn the sensual, provided that life is enjoyed with due restraint and moderation. In practice, however, this leads to a kind of tyranny of moderation in the context of which a good Protestant (in theory) indeed can enjoy life, but is (in practice) never moderate enough.

in the afterlife firmly remained its primary ideal of human existence. In this sense, happiness and joy coming from faith in God were mainly seen more as a joy of returning back to the right path to salvation and (hence) as an improvement over the salvation anxiety caused by the "deluded" Catholic idea of earning of merit. Even though these were certainly important initial leaps towards what will eventually become the modern experience of happiness, the Reformation (and counter-Reformation as its response), therefore, didn't bring fundamental transformations to the basic Christian formula of the relationship to the self.

Indeed, Foucault argues (1978, p. 116), the Reformation and counter-Reformation 'mark an important mutation and a schism in what might he called the traditional technology of the flesh[15]'. However, 'this did not rule out a certain parallelism in the Catholic and Protestant methods of examination of conscience and pastoral direction: procedures for analyzing "concupiscence" and transforming it into discourse'. The 'main features of both' the Protestant and Catholic churches, Foucault further explains (2000a, p. 243), are still 'an ensemble of truth obligations dealing with faith, books, dogma, and one dealing with truth, heart, and soul,' where 'access to truth cannot be conceived of without purity of the soul'.

Insofar as in the Protestant churches the refusal of the self and Christian self-deciphering in their essence remained, one form of anxiety was just replaced by another. Trying to amend the Catholic salvation anxiety through the doctrines of justification by faith and predestination, 'many Protestants' were now 'cast into deep despair at the thought that they were damned' (Thomas 2009, p. 232). An example of what could be called predestination anxiety[16] is the astrological doctor Richard Napier, who practiced in the early 17th century in England and who 'had over ninety patients who came to him because they doubted their prospects of salvation' (Thomas 2009, p. 232).

Next, we shall turn to the axis of power and analyze this turbulent period of Western history in light of power relations and struggles.

The Culmination of Struggles Around the Pastoral Power

As Von Greyerz (2008, p. 28) observes, 'the Reformation was an exclusively religious event in the beginning, but not so as it unfolded'. By looking 'at the carriers of the reformist movements in the 1520s,' he explains, 'it is not possible, in retrospect, to distinguish clearly between motives that were genuinely religious and those that were socioeconomic and political; that is true for both the cities and the countryside' (Von Greyerz 2008, p. 28). Or—informed by the more in-depth Foucauldian analysis of power relations in the medieval period—we should rather say that the Reformation movement was no doubt a struggle initiated by a doctrinal dispute,

[15] Which includes the refusal of (obligatory) confession by majority of the protestant churches.

[16] For more on Protestant 'religious despair,' see Stachniewski (1991).

which, however, had rapidly grown to a series of struggles over the pastoral power that were

> fundamentally struggles over who would actually have the right to govern men, and to govern them in their daily life and in the details and materiality of their existence; they were struggles over who has this power, from whom it derives, how it is exercised, the margin of autonomy for each, the qualification of those who exercise it, the limits of their jurisdiction, what recourse is possible against them, and what control is exercised over each other (Foucault 2007, p. 200).

Indeed, the period between the 13th and the 16th centuries in which we are focusing in this chapter was characterized by a particularly large intensity of struggles around the pastorate culminating in the spread of the Reformation movement and the Wars of Religion. The Reformation was, therefore, 'undoubtedly much more a great pastoral battle than a great doctrinal battle' (Foucault 2007, p. 200). In this sense, the main transformations of experience of sin induced by the Reformation movement described above (such as the return to scripture and to Augustine's refusal of free will; refusal of indulgences and obligatory confession and the refusal of hierarchy of the sacred) should be largely seen as the outcomes of pastoral struggles.

The culmination of pastoral struggles and the consequent transformations of the pastorate during the Reformation and counter-Reformation, however, did not bring the pastoral modality of power to an end because

> threatened by all these movements of counter-conduct, the Church tries to take them up and adapt them for its own ends, until the great separation takes place, the great division between the Protestant churches, which basically opt for a certain mode of re-implantation of these counter-conducts, and the Catholic Church, which tries to re-utilize them and re-insert them in its own system through the Counter Reformation (Foucault 2007, p. 282).

It, hence, follows 'that the two worlds or series of worlds that issue from the Reformation, that is to say, a Protestant world, or a world of Protestant churches and the counter-Reformation, were not worlds without a pastorate'. On the contrary, Foucault explains (2007, p. 200), 'What resulted from the Reformation was a formidable reinforcement of the pastorate in two different types'. On the one side, there was the 'Protestant type, or the type developed by different Protestant sects, with a meticulous pastorate, but one that was all the more meticulous as it was hierarchically supple,' and, on the other side, there was the 'counter-Reformation with a pastorate entirely brought back under control, a hierarchized pyramid, within a strongly centralized Catholic church'.

The First Steps Towards the Birth of Happiness

Above, we have seen that the Christian problematization of salvation, which lasted from the 5th to the 16th century, was fundamentally marked by original sin, which did not allow humans to find true bliss on earth. In our view, this experience of sin cannot be simply equated with the experience of happiness, which only emerged in the 17th and 18th centuries, when the ideal of human existence increasingly started to be pursued in the present life. In other words, we do not believe that the birth of happiness can be simply seen as a process of happiness descending down from heaven to earth because it was never up there in the first place. As we have seen in the discussion above, throughout the medieval period, heaven was associated with the concept of bliss [*beatitudo*] and not with the concept of happiness. Happiness was born in this world and primarily pertains to this world.

In the next chapter, we shall try to show that the birth of experience of happiness is largely connected with the intensification of the problematization of (good) feeling on earth, and the affirmation of everyday life, which emerged in the 14th and 15th centuries, for some time existed parallel to the problematization of salvation and eventually (since the beginning of the 17th century) started to slowly overshadow it. Let us explain this more thoroughly starting with semantics.

In the original Christian canon (and later also in medieval theological and scholastic writing), the word designating the ultimate ideal of human existence was the Latin expression *beati/beatitude*, which is a Vulgate translation of the Greek term *makarios*, which at least in the Christian tradition carried an exalted religious connotation. In virtually all of the European languages (except Welsh) the words happy and happiness on the other hand, have their origins in expressions with purely mundane connotations. They either came from the Indo-European root *fe*, whose original meaning is the contentment of a baby suckling at the breast (neo-latin languages—Italian, Spanish, Portuguese), or either from the word for luck, which was always a more mundane expression (the majority of other European languages). Following from such etymology, the word happy initially designated some type of (good) fortune, chance or fertility in the earthly realm. It was only around the 16th and 17th centuries that in the major European languages the word happiness also started to signify a pleasant and contented mental state (see Harper 2011).

Even though since the 18th century beati(tudo) started to be increasingly translated as happy(iness) in the official Christian canon[17], we agree with Kreeft (1992), who is extremely critical towards such translations, arguing that the two expressions are both etymologically and theologically different. And, in fact, in the late Middle Ages, still characterized by the experience of sin and the problematization of salvation, neither the word happy nor happiness were originally intended to directly replace the Latin expressions for beati or beatitudo. Rather, the word happiness emerged as a part of a new kind of problematization—the problematization of (good) feeling on earth. This can be most clearly seen in Luther (1545), who, when referring to joy and happiness (Glück) coming from our faith in God, is not using these terms in a direct connection to salvation in the afterlife, but is positioning them in the registry of mundane earthly experience. While for Luther true salvation (beatitudo) is still seen as pertaining to the afterlife, personal relief from the anxiety of salvation coming from deep faith in God opens up and affirms a certain degree of positive feeling on earth, which is not explicitly sacralized.

[17] In Chap. 6 we shall see that this way of translating beatitude is related to Christianity operating in the new context of the modern experience of happiness.

In this chapter, we have argued that not only the Reformation movement, but also the Renaissance before it, each in their own specific ways contributed to the start of the problematization of (good) human feeling in the present life. While in the case of the Renaissance, this development was mostly driven by an increased interest in man, the reengagement of ancient philosophers and further affirmation of rationality and free will, the Reformation reinforced the problematization of feeling mostly in connection with the rejection of the sacred and the affirmation of mundane life.

The emergence and increased use of the expressions happy and happiness can be certainly linked to this two new problematizations. However, in our view, neither the emergence of problematization of (good) feeling nor the verbal designations for happiness connected to it simply coincided with the birth of experience of happiness. Rather, the problematization of (good) feeling on earth for some time only co-existed with the preceding and still dominating problematization of salvation, until in the 17th century the former started to slowly but surely dominate over the latter. We believe that it is precisely this transformation (in which good feeling on earth in connection with the affirmation of mundane life starts becoming the primary ideal of human existence) that represents the first major development, which marks the birth of the modern experience of happiness. The second such major development, besides the ideal of human existence becoming increasingly positioned in this life, is that the ideal of human existence also becomes perceived as entirely achievable with human efforts.

These two major developments not only mark the birth of happiness, but also represent the two major characteristics or parameters of the modern experience of happiness, which at the same time also fundamentally distinguish it from the preceding experience of sin. In order for this decisive transformation to occur on a larger scale, however, first the idea of (original) sin had to be refused. Namely, being the constitutive part of the medieval Christian experience, the idea of (original) sin represented the main inhibition precluding the ideal of human existence to be positioned in this life. Furthermore, in spite of the gradual trend of reinforcement of free will underway since the 9th century, due to the idea of original sin it was still held that the ideal of human existence was not entirely achievable by human efforts alone.

The next chapter shall attempt to trace this decisive transformation of experience.

Chapter 6
The Birth of Modern Happiness

The Truth About Happiness

In the previous chapter, we have described two major currents of thought that have—still within the dominant problematization of salvation and each from a different angle—from the fourteenth to the sixteenth century started problematizing (good) human feeling in the present life. The crucial step towards the birth of modern happiness on the axis of truth was the fusion of these two currents of thought: a bringing together of Protestant affirmation of ordinary life with the ideas of human freedom and rationality intensified from the ninth century, reinforced by Aquinas and the Renaissance and culminating in the beginning of empiricism of Francis Bacon and Galileo Galilei. On the axis of truth, this fusion caused the problematization of (good) feeling on earth in connection with the affirmation of everyday life to start dominating over the problematization of salvation, resulting in a gradual transformation of experience of sin into the experience of happiness.

The early form of the convergence between the rationalist current and (the Protestant) current of affirmation of everyday life took shape in what is usually called Deism. 'Retaining something of the original theological outlook surrounding the affirmation of ordinary life' and combining it with the emphasis on rationality, Deism can be best understood as a kind of 'rationalist Christianity' (Taylor 2001, p. 234). One of its cardinal figures was John Locke, whose teachings had an immense influence on the whole development of the fusion between the affirmation of everyday life and rational employment of free will. By way of the atheist and naturalist turn in the eighteenth century, this fusion eventually led to the Enlightenment movement and, consequently, to the birth of the modern secular experience of happiness on the axis of truth (which will be described in the next chapter).

If it was crucial for the emergence of experience of happiness on the axis of truth that the ideal of human existence become increasingly connected to life on earth, an important aspect of the birth of happiness has to be associated with the erosion of original sin—the main hindrance, which, in the Christian experience of sin, didn't allow envisioning of such an ideal in the present life.

L. Zevnik, *Critical Perspectives in Happiness Research*,
DOI 10.1007/978-3-319-04403-3_6, © Springer International Publishing Switzerland 2014

God as the Foundation for Happiness on Earth

The seventeenth century was characterized by a sparkling discussion in the intellectual circles regarding the question of innate ideas in the human mind. Ancient philosophers, medieval theologians and the majority of influential thinkers of the time (including Descartes and leading Anglican divines) maintained that either nature or 'God, in his infinite goodness and wisdom, has inscribed in human minds innate principles that constitute the foundation of knowledge, both in practical and in theoretical matters' (Rickless 2007, p. 33). Locke's famous *Essay Concerning Human Understanding* was written as a frontal attack on such doctrines of innate ideas conceived by Locke as a position maintaining that 'there are in the Understanding certain innate Principles; some primary Notions, Koimai_mmoiai [common notions], Characters, as it were stamped upon the Mind of Man, which the Soul receives in its very first Being; and brings into the World with it' (Locke 1979, 1.2.1). Following from such a doctrine, according to Locke, Rickless explains (2007, p. 44), is 'that God (or Nature) is the author of innate principles' and that 'innate practical principles serve as a guide to human action'. In relation to happiness, this means that the main point of God having imprinted innate ideas on human minds 'is that humans might thereby come to know what can be known and recognize what needs to be done in order to achieve happiness' (Rickless 2007, p. 44).

Refusing the notion of innate ideas, Locke gives an altogether different answer to the question, 'What is it that determines the Will in regard to our Actions' (Locke 1979, 2.21). Inspired by a seventeenth-century French mathematician and priest, Pierre Gassendi, who aimed to develop a Christian system based on Epicurean philosophy, Locke 'adopts a hedonist theory' (Taylor 2001, p. 169). Rather than seeing humans as tending by nature towards the good, Locke argues that things 'are good or evil only in reference to pleasure or pain' (Locke 1979, 2.20.1). More specifically: 'Good and evil, present and absent, it is true, work upon the mind. But that which immediately determines the will, from time to time, to every voluntary action, is the uneasiness of desire' (Locke 1979, 2.21.33). Locke's (1979, 2.21.43) answer to what moves this uneasiness of desire is central to his understanding of happiness:

> If it be further asked, what tis moves desire? I answer happiness and that alone. Happiness and Misery are the names of two extremes, the utmost bound whereof we know not; tis what Eye hath not seen, Ear hath not heard, nor hath it entered into the Heart of Man to conceive [1 Cor. 2:9]. But of some degrees of both, we have very lively impressions, made by several instances of Delight and Joy on the one side and Torment and Sorrow on the other; which, for shortness sake, I shall comprehend under the names of Pleasure and Pain, there being pleasure and pain of the Mind, as well as the body… Happiness then in its full extent is the utmost Pleasure we are capable of, and Misery, the utmost Pain.

We can clearly see that the problematization of (good) feeling on earth that now takes the form of pleasure is central in Locke's understanding of the ideal of human existence that now becomes happiness. If one wants to achieve happiness, the cardinal ethical question to tackle, then, is how to achieve the utmost pleasure and avoid the utmost pain.

Counting on reason and the power of free will, Locke believes that the mind has 'a power to suspend the execution of any of its desires; and so all, one after another, is at liberty to consider the objects in them, examine them on all sides, and weigh them with others' (Locke 1979, 2.21.53). That is, based on empirical evidence, we can determine what is the greatest good and discover the way to seek it: 'A man may suspend the act of his choice from being determined for or against the thing proposed, till he has examined whether it be really of a nature, in itself and its consequences, to make him happy or not' (Locke 1979, 2.21.57). With his hedonist theory, Locke is, therefore, not simply arguing that there 'might be as many paths to happiness as there are pleasures of men' (McMahon 2006, p. 184). On the contrary, he believes that 'fashion and the common opinion have settled wrong notions, and education and custom ill habits, the just values of things misplaced, and palates of men corrupted' (Locke 1979, 2.21.71). However, given that there are no innate ideas in the mind, we have the possibility to 'remake ourselves in a more rational and advantageous fashion' (Taylor 2001, p. 170). In other words, 'Since we have a powerful drive toward happiness,' Wilson explains (2007, p. 401), moral steering for Locke 'often requires only the correction of false beliefs concerning what will make us happy'.

With his Protestant (Puritan) background, Locke saw the rational goals of such remaking in following the law laid down by God, which at times he also calls the Natural Law. God's or Natural Law in this sense is, therefore, 'not only what we ought to do morally, but it is also what conduces to our greatest happiness' (Taylor 2001, p. 171). The particular way in which Locke associates divine commands and human reason points to the fact that while being a hedonist, he was also a theological voluntarist:

> Moral good and evil … is only the conformity or disagreement of our voluntary action to some law, whereby good or evil is drawn on us, from the will and power of the law-maker, which good or evil, pleasure or pain, attending our observance or breach of the law by the decree of the lawmaker, is that we call reward and punishment (Locke 1979, 2.28.5).

Following from the logic of this hedonism, 'God's law is the law normative for us not because he is our creator or infinitely good, but because he proffers a totally credible threat of overwhelming retribution to the disobedient' (Taylor 2001, p. 235). In other words, Our pursuits of happiness 'are constrained only by what God (the Law of Nature) explicitly prohibits' (Wilson 2007, p. 401).

As Taylor (2001, p. 236) explains, Locke's 'amalgam of voluntarism and hedonism' enables him 'to see the Law of Nature both as Divine command and as the dictate of reason: The reason in question is instrumental. Once we see that we are creatures of an omnipotent lawgiver, the rational thing is to obey'. Locke drives his 'rationalized Christianity' even further by arguing that 'not only that obeying God is the (instrumentally) rational thing to do but even that (theoretical) reason can discern the content of God's will' (Taylor 2001, p. 236). This means that 'although we in fact learn of God's law through revelation, we could in principle reach similar conclusions by reason alone' (Taylor 2001, p. 236): 'God, like a super-player in a game of rational choice, instrumentalizes our instrumental reason by giving us a law which brings us into line with his purpose of general conservation' and well-being (Taylor 2001, p. 236). While in the Protestant vision of affirmation of everyday life 'it was a matter of living worshipfully for God, now it is becoming a question of living rationally' (Taylor 2001, p. 242).

In the Deist linking of reason and religion, 'God's purposes fully respect humans' autonomous reason' (Taylor 2001, p. 245), and 'the exercise of rationality is the way we take part in God's plan' (Taylor 2001, p. 242). With the rational logic driving 'towards rational transparency,' there are no more places for mystery in such rationalized religion (Taylor 2001, p. 245). The book written by Toland (who was Locke's contemporary) entitled *Christianity Not Mysterious* (1702) is a very revealing example of this general trend.

According to Lowe (2002, p. 17), Locke's position on innate ideas has been predominantly motivated by two reasons. The first was connected with the fact that 'in Britain, as opposed to the continent of Europe, the new science of the seventeenth century had already been given a more empiricist cast by the writings of Francis Bacon (1561–1626) on the one hand, and by the scientific work of such experimentalists as Hooke, Boyle and Newton on the other'. Locke's hostility towards the doctrine of innate ideas, however, was not only related to the danger he saw in it to the freedom of thought and inquiry in the field of science, but also in matters of ethics, religion and politics. 'By contrast to the quietest Descartes,' Lowe observes (2002, p. 18), 'Locke was a champion of individual liberty and rights at a time when these were, in Britain at least, enjoying a precarious flowering'. In this sense, he saw the doctrine of innate ideas also as 'inherently prone to exploitation by conservative and reactionary forces, because it is only too easy to appeal to supposedly God-given principles of morality and religion to attempt to silence challenges to prevailing authority and interests' (Lowe 2002, p. 18).

One such principle was also the notion of original sin, which Locke's refusal of the doctrine of innate ideas ultimately helped to erase[1]. According to the traditional Christian perspective of salvation, original sin resulted in humanity losing the capacities for achieving true bliss on earth and stained humans with lust and concupiscence. While in this sense desire was a consequence of original sin and had to be neutralized, Locke saw the human desire for pleasure and the seeking to avoid pain (i.e. the problematization of (good) feeling) not as 'a failing but an unalterable feature' of human make-up. For Locke and also other Deists, Taylor explains (2001, p. 242), 'Our fear of endless pain and our desire for unspeakable joys, is not evil. It is made by God and therefore good'. What English empiricism, therefore, 'introduces—let's say, roughly, with Locke—, and doubtless for the first time in Western philosophy,' Foucault explains, 'is a subject who is not so much defined by his freedom, or by the opposition of soul and body, or by the presence of a source or core of concupiscence marked to a greater or lesser degree by the Fall or sin, but who appears in the form of a subject of individual choices' (Foucault 2008, p. 376). Along with original sin, the idea of grace and divine intervention also loses its meaning: 'If the good of man that God calls to becomes more and more available to human rational scrutiny, it also becomes more and more encompassable with hu-

[1] A more indirect refusal of original sin could also be found in the ideas of the so-called natural theologians writing in roughly the same time as Locke (such as John Ray (1691) and William Derham (1711)) who argued that God as the Devine Architect created a providential order designed for the harmonious benefit and well-being of its inhabitants, a notion that was -as we shall see- also adopted by Locke and other Deists.

man powers' (Taylor 2001, p. 245). In Locke's words, this simply means that 'men's happiness or misery is most part of their own making' (Locke 1996, p. 10).

Following from this, the Deist convergence (especially Locke) can be seen as the final defeat of the radical Augustinian current of the refusal of free will, which we had traced since its birth in the time of the Pelagian polemic to its revival in the Reformation movement. Somewhat paradoxically, Deism, therefore, subverted the Protestant current of refusal of free will, out of which the affirmation of everyday life, one of its central components, had emerged. Namely, above, we have seen that one of the central Protestant theological points emphasized behind the affirmation of everyday life was the affirmative and cathartic embracing of human nature and its limitations. Refusing the Catholic ascent up the ladder of being, 'The Reformers stressed the ungodly motivation of pride that led people to try to transcend the ordinary lay condition' (Taylor 2001, p. 242). Instead, they argued, we should humbly accept the nature God has given us. According to Taylor (2001, p. 242), the Deist acceptance of hedonism, 'the fact that we are impelled by nature to maximize pleasure,' can be seen in a similar light: 'Rather than aspire to a self-abnegating altruism for which we are not made, we should accept our nature and fulfill God's purpose in it'.

Insofar as Locke and other Deists and natural theologians doubt that either nature or God has inscribed certain innate ideas (such as original sin) on human minds, it, hence, also follows that there cannot be anything inherent in the human nature that would inhibit the pursuit of happiness both in this world and in the life to come. While within the Christian experience of sin it was impossible for humans to achieve the ultimate ideal of existence on earth, now every human being has the potential to achieve happiness with his own efforts already in the present life.

In this sense, Deism and natural theology along the line of affirmation of everyday life transposed the universalizing message of Christianity from the universal sinfulness to the idea of a universal providential order created by the merciful God for the common benefit and happiness of all of its inhabitants both in heaven and on earth. That is, rather than in grace and divine intervention, in their view, the goodness of God 'manifests itself in the beneficence of the regular order of things' (Taylor 2001, p. 272). In this sense, 'It is not the fallenness of the world but its perfection of design which now becomes crucial. People need not be saved from a reigning disorder, but rather to learn to conform properly to the design of things' (Taylor 2001, p. 272).

Following from this, Deists also did not see the individual pursuit of happiness as an egoistic and self-centered activity. On the contrary, they believed that living in line with the divine providential order can be 'industrious and rational in meeting our own needs and hence, through the improvements which result help to meet the needs of others' (Taylor 2001, p. 239). Due to such a combination of self-service and beneficence based on divine providential order, Deism (especially Hutcheson) prepared the ground for the Enlightenment ideal of harmony of interests, which culminated in a utilitarian philosophy.

By refusing original sin and by emphasizing rationality and earthly pleasure, the Deist convergence and the natural theology constituted an important part of the process that caused the problematization of good feeling on earth (now understood as pleasure and happiness) to start replacing the problematization of salvation. The birth of happiness in the seventeenth century was not, however, only limited to intellectual circles of Deist philosophers. While Deism certainly helped to articulate the emerging modern (religious) experience of happiness on the axis of truth, it was basically a part of a much larger trend.

As McMahon notes (2006, p. 190), 'The final two decades of the seventeenth century witnessed an explosion of works on happiness'. In London bookstores, one could find books like *A Persuasive to a Holy Life from the Happiness that Attends it Both in this World, and in the World to Come; The Way to Health, Long Life and Happiness; England's Happiness Improved; An Infallible way to get Riches, Encrease Plenty, and Promote Pleasure, etc.* (Mcmahon 2006, p. 191).

The happiness trend could also be increasingly observed in art. An illuminating example is Tate's adaptation of Shakespeare's tragedy King Lear in 1681, 'which sought to improve upon the original by, among other things, giving the play a happy ending' (McMahon 2006, p. 192). Even more than the idea itself, it was revealing that the 'adaptation proved tremendously appealing to contemporary audiences, holding the stage in preference to the original well into the nineteenth century' (McMahon 2006, p. 192). Theatre was not alone in following the happiness trend, as in poetry of this period one can also observe 'the consolidation of a more general image of the happy man, who succeeds in living his days happily until the end' (Mcmahon 2006, p. 192).

By far, the most convincing sign of a wider shift away from experience of sin to the modern experience of happiness emerging in the seventeenth century can be found in the official Church, which still maintained a major influence on the common folk. According to Thomas (2009, p. 226), "In the late seventeenth and early eighteenth centuries, much was said by Anglican divines about the 'pleasantness' of religion and the daily happiness it could bring to those who practiced it". In 1675, for example (15 years before Locke's Essay Concerning Human Understanding), Richard Allestree who was a leading English Royalist divine published his Arts of Contentment, a book that went through over 20 editions, remaining in print until the nineteenth centuries, which, in simple words, captured the tenor of his age. While Allestree (1677) acknowledged that 'every man would have happiness,' he was also quick to remark that most of the people lose themselves in 'blind pursuits'. Being a man of the Church, he naturally saw a solution in following God who is 'happy in himself' and who can show us 'a more certain, a more compendious way to acquire what we grasp after'. According to Allestree (1677), in the Gospel everybody can find 'a plain, a safe, nay a pleasant path, as much superior both in the ease of the way, and in the end to which it leads, as heaven is to Canaan'. In contrast to the Israelites, however, Allestree argues (1677), we need not wander in 'wild pursuits' to find happiness in the promised land; 'we may form it within our own breasts'. For Allestree (1677), the potentiality for happiness already in the present life, therefore, lies within us all and Christianity is the only true beacon that shows the right way and as such represents 'certainly the most excellent, the most compendious art of happy living' in which 'all the lines of wordly happiness are concentrated'.

In the widely read works of the official Church figures such as Allestree, it is therefore possible to identify a crucial development slowly taking its root even within the official Christian religion—one that not only promises ultimate bliss in the afterlife, but clearly also starts employing the Gospel to improve the human condition already in the present life[2]. In the context of the modern experience of happiness, (Christian) religion eventually comes down to mainly performing this role.

As McMahon (2006, p. 195) observes, the general forces that had worked to create a space for the birth of happiness in England were at work abroad, too:

> in Scotland and Ireland, in the American colonies, and on the European continent, influential voices were beginning to draw similar conclusions from the combined precedents of Renaissance Humanism and innovative Christian theology, imagining a place for pleasure and felicity on earth. As increasing numbers began to think beyond the boundaries of sin, the scope for Western happiness widened considerably.

In the seventeenth century, the problematization of good feeling/pleasure in connection with the affirmation of everyday life (or in short the problematization of happiness[3]) slowly but surely started to dominate over the problematization of salvation, producing a wider shift from the ideal of existence focused on eternal bliss in heaven and afterlife to the ideal of pursuing happiness (through pleasure) in the present life. This development can already be seen as the beginning of a purely modern experience of happiness on the axis of truth, which differs from the preceding experience of sin in almost all major aspects except in retaining certain elements of Christian divinity. While salvation in the afterlife is still regarded as the final goal, there is a clear trend (among the clergymen, laymen and (Deist) philosophers alike) of religion being increasingly understood primarily as a foundation for happiness on earth. This trend will become even more obvious in the eighteenth century when even 'otherwise orthodox members of the church were penning treatises with popular titles like *I want to Be Happy, The School of Happiness,* and *The Theory of Happiness, or the Art of Rendering Oneself So*' (McMahon 2006, p. 204). It is revealing that in line with this trend in numerous religious books and even in the Christian canon, the word beatitude (blessedness) characterizing the ideal of human existence within the Christian problematization of salvation eventually started being translated as happiness, de facto implying that the modern form of Christianity is actually closer to the modern experience of happiness rather than to the medieval experience of sin. And, in fact, according to Thomas (2009, p. 267), although the church influence on society was still considerable

> in practice, most of the population implicitly took a more secular view: they cherished life for its own sake, not merely as a preliminary to some future state. Highly aware of the satisfactions which they could hope to find in their work and their possessions, the affection of their friends and families, and the respect of their peers, they increasingly sought fulfillment in their daily existence.

---

[2] Here we should note that this innovation was did not go completely unquestioned. There were some conservative and reactionary churchmen such as Edmund Calamy (1662), who still vigorously emphasized the old Christian vision of salvation.

[3] From the point when the problematization of good feeling/pleasure and the affirmation of everyday life become firmly consolidated and dominant, also a shorter (but wider) expression can also be used: the problematization of happiness.

Insofar as this early form of happiness is still retaining certain religious elements, we shall call it the religious experience of happiness. In the broadest sense, it could be seen as a basic model for the majority of all future religious experiences of happiness in Western culture that range from the various expressions of Christian religiosity to the so-called new-age spirituality emerging in the second half of the twentieth century[4].

In addition to the religious experience of happiness in development since the seventeenth century, in the eighteenth century a secular experience of happiness also emerged as part of the continuation of the process of the birth of happiness in Western culture. Its introduction is largely connected to the secularization processes catalyzed by the Enlightenment movement.

Enlightenment and the Birth of Modern Secular Happiness

In 1705, the Dutch preacher Johannes Aalstius argued in his general introduction to Christian ethics that the new radicalism, and especially Spinozism,[5] 'overturns the entire structure of divinely ordained morality' (Aalstius 1705 in Israel 2001, p. 5). Were such developments to gain wide acceptance, he further warned, 'mankind would in the future concern itself only with individual happiness in this life' (Aalstius 1705 in Israel 2001, p. 5). As it turned out, his predictions (at least regarding the pursuit of happiness exclusively in this life) were right.

Sweeping across Europe since the second half of the seventeenth century, the Enlightenment movement started to 'challenge everything inherited from the past—not just commonly received assumptions about mankind, society, politics, and the cosmos, but also the veracity of the Bible and the Christian faith or indeed any faith' (Israel 2001, p. 4). Whereas before 1650 confessional differences and conflicts were at the centre of concern, by the 1680s an increasing number of French, Dutch, German and English writers began to note that 'the main issue now was the escalating contest between faith and incredulity' (Israel 2001, p. 4). The rationalization and secularization process 'rapidly overthrew theology's age-old hegemony in the world of study and 'slowly but surely eradicated magic and belief in the supernatural from Europe's intellectual culture' (Israel 2001, p. 4). In practice, many ordinary people also followed the trend of intellectual revolution. According to Israel (2001, p. 6), proofs that 'new ideas were rapidly transforming attitudes and beliefs throughout society' were 'abundantly evident on every side and in every part of

[4] We are not implying that so-called new-age spirituality also worships Christian God, which in fact most of the numerous new-age approaches don't. Rather we would like to suggest that many new-age approaches share this basic model of accepting a certain divine, higher principle or force, which a person has to take into account or follow in order to pursue happiness in the present life.

[5] We are on the same page with Israel (2001, p. 159) that Spinoza indeed had no rival as the chief progenitor and author of the main radical enlightenment ideas of 'eliminating divine Providence and governance of the world' that have culminated in 'the Naturalistic, materialist, one-substance' system of thought characteristic of the Enlightenment.

Europe'. As Seckedorff, for example, observed in as early as 1685 (in Israel 2001, p. 6), this growing trend among ordinary folk included mocking the holy scripture, rejecting heaven and hell, doubting the immortality of the soul and questioning the existence of Satan, demons and spirits.

Eighteenth-century Europe was, hence, increasingly witnessing 'the regression of belief in God, and even more, the decline in the practice of religion, to the point where from being central to the whole life of Western societies, public and private, this has become sub-central, one of many private forms of involvement which some people indulge in' (Taylor 2001, p. 309). Logically, such processes had important consequences for the experience of happiness, which slowly but surely became a central goal of human existence from the second half of the seventeenth century onwards.

Although the current Deist and the accompanying wider social and religious developments have already quite firmly re-orientated the focus of the ideal of human existence to gravitate more to the earthly realm, the religious experience of happiness that these developments had produced still included the ideas of heaven, divine providence and governance of the world. Enlightenment, on the other hand, has stripped happiness completely clear of its religious outlook, producing the secular modern experience of happiness, which is—as we shall see—manifested in two main modes.

Holbach's *Christianity Unveiled* (1761) is perhaps one of the most directs attacks on the old Christian tradition and, at the same time, a clear paving of the way towards the modern secular vision of happiness, which, in its basic formula—with certain developments of course—still persists today. In the typical Enlightenment spirit, Holbach's critical reflection of Christianity is set up as an examination of whether it (along with Judaism and also other religions) can contribute to individual and communal happiness. Holbach (1761, Chap. 11) puts all the major aspects of Christian religion, from its mysteries, dogmas, rites, and ceremonies to priesthood, morality and politics, to the test of discerning reason and vigorously concludes that Christianity in all its facets contributes only to the 'destruction of human happiness'. In his view, Christian religion 'can be advantageous only to ignorant and vicious princes, who are desirous to reign over slaves, and who, in order to strip and tyrannize over them with impunity, form a league with the priesthood, whose function it has ever been to deceive in the name of heaven' (Holbach 1761, Chap. 16).

For the radical Enlightenment thinkers like Holbach, Voltaire, Diderot and La Metrrie, Christianity and along with it its illusory ideal of human existence envisaged as salvation in heaven stand as obstacles to the potential of true improvement of the human condition only achievable in the form of happiness on Earth. 'Hell is no more; tis Heaven now on earth …,' observed another Enlightenment philosopher Claude-Adrien Helvetius (in McMahon 2006, p. 199) in his poem *Happiness*. In the Christian perspective, true bliss was only accessible in the afterlife. The Enlightenment perspective, on the contrary, refuses the possibilities of life beyond this world and sees the potential for true happiness as something only pertaining to life on Earth. Before, Holbach argues (1761, Chap. 16), people were led to expect 'happiness from chimeras' merely because they were 'forbidden to seek for it from realities'. While due to original sin it was held before that humans were not able to achieve true bliss in the present life, now human beings are perceived as intended by nature to pursue and achieve happiness exclusively in this world.

The Enlightenment philosophers agreed with the Deist perspective in considering the pursuit of happiness as a universal possibility (which is entirely achievable by human effort), but they diverged in their understanding of the foundations of this universal possibility. In this sense, the Deist understanding of God as the source and the bestower of happiness through the creation of the divine providential order is replaced by nature herself who—personified in Holbach's (1966) *Systeme de la nature*—is calling to us humans: 'O you, says she, who, according to the inclination that I give you, tend towards happiness in every instant of your existence, do not resist my sovereign law. Work towards your happiness; Enjoy without fear, be happy' (Holbach 1966, p. 3). As for those still clinging to the divine, the voice of nature exclaims,

> In vain, o superstitious one! do you seek your well-being beyond the limits of the universe where my hand has placed you. In vain do you ask it of these inexorable fantoms which your imagination wishes to establish on my eternal throne … in vain do you trust in these capricious deities whose beneficence sends you into ecstasy; while they fill your sojourn with dread, with wailing, with illusions. Therefore dare to free yourself from the yoke of this religion, my proud rival, that does not recognize my laws. In my dominion reigns liberty … Come back then, child, deserter, come back to nature! She will console you, she will chase from your heart these fears which overwhelm you, these worries which tear at you, these outbursts which agitate you, these hatreds which separate you from man whom you should love (Holbach 1966, p. 3).

No wonder, then, McMahon observes (2006, p. 200) with the help of Mauzi (1994) and Hazard (1969), that 'no previous age wrote so much on the subject or so often. In France, Britain, and the Low Countries, in Germany, Italy, and the United States, disquisitions on happiness poured from the presses: reflections on happiness, treatises on happiness, systems of happiness, discourses, essays, sketches, and epistles'. And as Hazard (1969) notes further, in all major European cities, the College of Nobles even organized a lecture series on the theme 'Man's Happiness Here Below'. The Enlightenment period, hence, further intensified the problematization of (good) feeling and happiness already initiated by the Deist convergence of the affirmation of everyday life and the rational employment of free will. Following from its secular perspective, the pursuit of happiness for the first time became completely independent from the divine and exclusively limited to the earthly realm.

Similar to the Deist view that had preceded it, the Enlightenment perspective is also starting from the problematization of good feeling/pleasure on earth, which implies that people desire happiness and pleasure and strive to avoid pain. From their secular views, however, it follows that in order to maximize happiness, we cannot rely on a divine providential order inherently designed for the common good and happiness of its inhabitants[6]. Instead, as Enlightenment thinkers argued, we have to

---

[6] The idea of the divine providential order was not only questioned theoretically, but also satirized in works such as Voltaire's Candide (2006) and Samuel Johnson's Rasselas (1805), which were symptomatically both published in 1759 after the catastrophic Lisbon earthquake.

look at the world and at our own natures, 'as a neutral domain, which we have to understand in order to master it, and whose causal relations we have to make use of in order to produce the greatest amount of happiness' (Taylor 2001, p. 321). The crucial judgment for any action, then, cannot be based on the rational understanding of a pre-existing law (like Locke's Law of God), but on the rational understanding of the consequences of this action. Following from this enlightenment, ethics were purely based on utility, where the principle of utility corresponded to 'that principle which approves or disapproves of every action whatsoever, according to the tendency which it appears to have to augment or diminish the happiness of the party whose interest is in question: or, what is the same thing in other words, to promote or to oppose that happiness[7]' (Bentham 2000, Chap. 1). In this sense, the inherent human inclination to maximize pleasure and avoid pain is not understood solely in terms of the motives for human action, but also constitutes the principal moral standard of right and wrong.

Even though such utilitarian understanding of happiness is usually associated with the English philosophical school of utilitarianism (headed by Jeremy Bentham and John Stuart Mill), it was in fact—at least implicitly—common to almost all Enlightenment thinkers[8].

For the majority of early Enlightenment thinkers, the central part of the doctrine about human happiness was also the view 'that there was a potential harmony of interests between human beings' (Taylor 2001, p. 330), which was—as we have seen above—already anticipated by Deism (most prominently by Hutcheson). Contrary to Deism, however, the secularist Enlightenment thinkers didn't see the basis for such harmony of interests in the already existent divine providential order created by God for the well-being of its inhabitants. Instead, they believed that men should efficiently use natural resources and properly (e. i. rationally) organize society so that 'the felicity of each would consist with and even conduce to the felicity of all' (Taylor 2001, p. 330). In doing so—of course—they would have to take into account the principle of utility and the natural causalities that govern the play of pleasure and pain. 'No longer was,' Porter explains (1996, p. 11), 'the Universe a pious mystery, pervaded by occult powers and spiritual destinies; it was a machine that could be taken to bits, put together again, mended, altered and improved'.

Above, we have seen that for the Enlightenment philosophers, the principle of maximizing pleasure and minimizing pain constitutes the main moral standard of

[7] Bentham even goes so far as to argue that pleasure and pain in fact constitute the root of all psychological entities: 'Among all the several species of psychological entities… the two which are as it were the roots, the main pillars or foundations of all the rest, the matter of which all the rest are composed—or the receptacles of that matter, which so ever may be the physical image, employed to give aid, if not existence to conception, will be, it is believed… seen to be, Pleasures and Pains. Of these, the existence is matter of universal and constant experience. Without any of the rest, these are susceptible of,—and as often as they come unlooked for, do actually come into, existence: without these, no one of all those others ever had, or ever could have had, existence' (Bentham in Schofield 2006, p. 30).

[8] In Das Kapital Marx (1982, p. 758) for example regarded English utilitarian philosophy only as a dull reproduction of the preceding French enlightenment philosophers.

right and wrong. Taking also the idea of harmony of interests into account, it then follows that this principle of utility holds not only for the individual subject, but also for the collective subject. Hence, the famous Bentham's declaration in Fragment of Government: 'It is the greatest happiness[9] of the greatest number that is the measure of right and wrong' (Bentham 1969, p. 45). Following from the connection between happiness and the idea of harmony of interests, Enlightenment thinkers frequently problematized the dimension of collective happiness, which was often referred to as public happiness (see, e.g., Chastellux 1774).

But how did the Enlightenment thinkers conceive of harmony of interest without the foundation of morality in the divine providential order? First, they connected benevolence with (scientific) reason, which resulted in the idea that 'disengaged rationality seems to separate us from our own narrow, egoistic standpoint and make us capable of grasping the whole picture' (Taylor 2001, p. 331). Insofar as we are, thus, 'no longer imprisoned in the self, we are free to pursue the universal good' (Taylor 2001, p. 331). And second, 'in giving central significance to sensual pleasure and pain, and in challenging all the different conceptions of order, the utilitarians made it possible for the first time to put the relief of suffering, human but also animal, at the centre of the social agenda' (Taylor 2001, p. 331). This is possible, they maintained, because in the perfect situation, by using the power of reason, 'everyone would understand and act in full cognizance of this harmony, that each would seek happiness in what made for general happiness' (Taylor 2001, p. 330).

The importance attributed by the majority of Enlightenment thinkers to the moral dimension of happiness that manifested as the idea of harmony of interest becomes obvious when one considers that secular views can also serve as a basis for quite a different moral outlook. Namely, if pleasure and happiness are seen as the ultimate goals of human existence that is not founded on any divine order created for the beneficence of all its inhabitants, but purely on natural causal relations, then materialism and naturalism can also lead to a position of purely amoral egoistic hedonism. Even in the progressive spirit of the eighteenth century, few people dared to publicly employ the notions of materialism and naturalism so radically. Arousing great controversy amongst their contemporaries and suspicion by the authorities, Julien Offray de La Mettrie and later Marquis de Sade were the most famous of the lot.

La Mettrie studied medicine under Boerhaave, the most famous medical man of the time in Europe, 'which shaped the initial phase of his career as a writer and philosophe' (Israel 2001, p. 704). Following from his medical background, his first philosophical work was a scientific study of the soul with a suggestive title L'Historie naturelle de l'ame, in which he radicalized the materialism of his medical teacher and combined it with elements of Spinozist monism, dangerously hinting that 'what is called the soul is simply the sum total of its bodily parts, the final product of the interaction of matter' (McMahon 2006, p. 224). Threatening to erode

[9] While this famous phrase is commonly associated with Bentham, McMahon explains (2006, p. 212), 'He was merely reiterating what was already a widespread eighteenth-century conviction'. In fact, the "proto-variations" of the phrase were already employed by thinkers such as Hutchenson, Leibnitz, Beccaria and Helvetius (McMahon 2006, p. 212).

the centuries-old Western dualist conception of body and soul, the book caused turbulent outcry in France. The police seized all copies from the bookshops and La Mettrie had to flee to the Netherlands.

In exile, he produced his greatest work, L'Homme machine, in which he 'attempts to explain man's nature and his behavior in purely materialist terms, claiming that medical experience proves the different states of the soul are always linked to those of the body' (Israel 2001, p. 705). In this sense, La Mettrie understands human beings as nothing other than a natural machine, 'a self-winding machine, a living representation of perpetual motion' (La Mettrie 1994, p. 32). L'Homme machine was excessive even for the Dutch, known for their long tradition of tolerance. La Mattrie had to flee again. This time, he found refuge at the court of the freethinking Prussian king, Frederick the Great, where he spent the remaining 3 years of his short but intensive life further glorifying sensualism both in words and even more so in his actions.

Already from the naturalist system in L'Homme machine, it follows that happiness 'must begin by acknowledging frankly what we are—material beings, sophisticated animals, complex machines' (McMahon 2006, p. 226), unstoppably driven by the natural imperative for pleasure. Based on this assumption, McMahon explains (2006, p. 228), all of La Mettrie's subsequent works (*The System of Epicurus, The art of Enjoying oneself, The school of sensual pleasure, The Anti Seneca, The discourse on Happiness*) basically employed the same happiness formula; namely, that happiness lays 'in pleasure, in pleasure alone, and all who suggested otherwise were enemies of humanity, charlatans, or both'. For La Mettrie, 'purely and simply, pleasure was an affair of the organs—a matter of the senses, the sensation of matter. We should seek it any way we can' (McMahon 2006, p. 228).

While the majority of other Enlightenment thinkers also advocated pleasure and happiness as the cardinal human goal, they still maintained that the individual human tendency to maximize pleasure has to be synchronized with the common good (i.e. greatest happiness for the greatest numbers). Insofar as this also implies that our individual pursuit of happiness is not, as the Deist thinker Adam Smith (2002, p. 255) puts it, 'disturbing in any respect the happiness of our neighbor,' the rational idea of harmony of interests also dictates that either rational individuals themselves or—in case they are not capable of doing so—the government has to bound the manifestation of the innate and possibly egoistic drive for pleasure.

Refusing all such rational internal or external inhibitions to the unstoppable human drive for pleasure, La Mettrie and later also de Sade, on the contrary, demonstrated both in writing end even more so with their lives an entirely different mode of the modern secular experience of happiness. From the radical hedonist perspective, the idea of harmonious public happiness is far too idealistic and repressive, ignoring the empirical evidence of humans as instinctive pleasure machines. As a consequence, the utilitarian ideal of the greatest happiness for the greatest numbers is an illusion only conceivable in theory.

While for the dominant enlightenment current advocating the idea of harmony of interest, individuals have to rationally steer their drive for pleasure (i.e. rational hedonism), La Mettrie (in McMahon 2006, p. 229) sees reason, rather, as something that 'freezes the imagination and chases pleasure away'. Here, we have to note that La Mettrie is not completely abandoning reason—after all, he was writing scientific books. According to his study of the human machine driven by pleasure, however, it follows that reason has to be subordinated to the 'despotism of pleasure' (La Mettrie in Mcmahon 2006, p. 229).

La Mettrie (in Mcmahon 2006, p. 228), hence, radicalized the enlightenment hedonism and materialism to the extreme point of completely refusing morality and the common good on account of individual pleasure and happiness: 'It is thus very clear that with respect to happiness, good and evil are in themselves indifferent. The one who receives more satisfaction from doing evil will be happier than whoever receives less from doing good… Happiness is individual and particular, and may be found in the absence of virtue and even in crime'. That is, our egoistic pursuit for sensual gratification cannot be bound by any external or internal inhibition like law or morality. In addition, according to La Mettrie, happiness being individual and particular also means that happiness is not a priori bound to any specific range of experience (i.e. what is commonly perceived as agreeable), but can encompass the whole spectrum of human experience. He writes in *L'Anti-Seneque, ou Discours sur le bonheur* (La Mattrie in McMahon 2006, p. 228),

> May profane enjoyment and sensual indulgence, those two lubricious rivals, succeed each other in turn, melting you in pleasures, while making your soul as sticky and lascivious as your body. When you are spent, drink, eat, sleep, dream. If you insist on thinking on occasion, at least do so amidst two vines, sipping the pleasure of the present moment, or savoring the desire in store for you during the hour to come. Finally, if not content to outdo yourself in the great art of sensual pleasures, and if debauchery and dissolution are to your taste, perhaps filth and infamy will be more to your liking. Wallow in slime like a pig, and you will be happy in their fashion.

Apart from his written works, La Mettrie's radical hedonistic position also poured from his existence. He was supposedly a sensualist and bon vivant who openly and without reservation indulged in myriad sensual pleasures. La Mettrie, therefore, demonstrated both in theory and practice that the modern secular experience of happiness is marked by this irrational/Dionysian/instinctive drive for egoistic pleasure, which according to him cannot and/or should not be rationally curtailed.

Believing in the power of disengaged reason that in their view enables humans to act beyond their narrow selfish interest, it is not surprising, then, that even the most radical Enlightenment figures such as Voltaire, Diderot and Holbach vigorously condemned both his excessive theories and life. 'Dissolute, impudent, a flatterer, a buffoon,… died as he ought to have lived… killed by the ignorance that he professed,' Diderot observed (in McMahon 2006, p. 222), years after La Mettrie's death allegedly[10] caused by overeating and indigestion of pate de faisan aux truffes (pheasant paste). Even more so than his existential decadence, his Enlightenment contemporaries were appalled by his philosophy of purely egoistic hedonism: 'We are assured that there have been philosophers and atheists who have denied the distinction between virtue and vice, and who have preached debauchery and licence in

[10] The reasons for La Mettrie's death still haven't been completely disclosed as various theories and reports exist.

their morals. The author who has recently published L'Homme Machine has argued concerning morals like a frenzied madman' (Holbach in Taylor 2001, p. 334).

The reasons for the vigorous criticism of La Mettrie by his contemporaries were not only related to the fact that his vision of happiness was in direct conflict with their idea of harmony of interest, but also because his egoistic and immoral hedonism was based on the same naturalism and materialism that they themselves so eagerly professed. After all, even the advocates of the Enlightenment idea of harmony of interest readily recognized the drive for pleasure as an integral part of the modern secular experience of happiness. The fundamental disagreement between the proponents of the two modes of secular happiness concerned the understanding of what role this immanent human drive ought to play in their respective visions of human happiness. The harsh theoretical and moral attacks on La Metrrie alone point to the fact that the utilitarian enlightenment thinkers believed that the instinctive drive for egoistic pleasure is something that stands in the way of the public happiness based on the harmony of interest and, hence, has to be directed and restrained.

In addition to the modern religious experience of happiness that emerged in the seventeenth century, the process of the birth of happiness that continued well into the eighteenth century has also produced a secular experience of happiness, which conjoins two conflicting aspects. Spawned by the Enlightenment movement, both modes of the secular experience of happiness are based on materialistic and naturalistic views.

On the one hand, we have the dominant rationalistic-utilitarian mode that promotes public happiness, which, through the idea of harmony of interest, encompasses individual and communal happiness based on the principle of utility. On the other hand, we have the amoral mode of egoistic hedonism that advocates unrestrained expression of the individual's instinctive drive for pleasure.

There is no doubt that on the axis of truth the rationalistic-utilitarian mode was vastly dominant in terms of the sheer number of Enlightenment thinkers and their influence on the development of Western societies. The notorious marquise de Sade, who, towards the end of the eighteenth century and in the beginning of the nineteenth, in many respects drew from, lived by and further developed La Metrrie's vision of radical hedonism (and also d'Holbach's naturalism and materialism) was only an exception within this general trend.

The utilitarian vision of happiness advocating a certain restraint of the human drive for pleasure dominated not only theoretically, but also morally, politically and institutionally. This does not mean, however, that in practice the egoistic/irrational drive for pleasure diagnosed and pursued by La Metrrie and de Sade ceased to lurk in the depths of the Western subject of happiness. On the contrary, we believe that to a large extent it is precisely through the tension between the rationalistic-utilitarian mode and the amoral hedonist mode that the modern secular happiness is constituted on all axes of experience.

So let us now examine how, based on the dynamic between the two aspects of the secular experience of happiness, the dominant enlightenment current envisaged the path that, in their view, humanity should take in order to achieve (public) happiness and the improvement of the human condition on earth.

The (Infinite) Progress Towards Individual and Public Happiness

Insofar as they believed that both individual and public happiness cannot rely on a pre-existing providential order and, thus, ought to be pursued entirely by human effort, the mainstream enlightenment current intrinsically connected their utilitarian ideal of human happiness with scientific, technological, individual, social, political and economic progress. As Porter (1996, p. 12) explains, eighteenth-century thinkers 'developed from such assumption a fierce championing of individualism, a vindication of independence, the right of self-determination, self-improvement and happiness'.

As Kant (1784) proclaimed later in the century in his answer to the question 'What is enlightenment?' the motto of Enlightenment was *Sapere aude*—dare to know. Glorifying the power of reason, Enlightenment thinkers were confident that only better understanding and the development of knowledge about the world, the natural laws, man and human laws can truly improve the human condition and bring the greatest happiness for the greatest numbers. In addition, science and technology, philosophy, political theory and (moral) education were perceived as the cornerstones of progress towards the improvement of the human condition on earth.

The rapidly developing science and technology based on empirical observation pioneered by Bacon and Galilei and further developed by experimentalists and innovators such as Hooke, Boyle and Newton gradually started improving material conditions in Europe. Advances in agricultural productivity and improvements in livestock breeding meant that Europeans ate more and better than before. With superior nutrition and advances in medicine and hygiene, people were also less susceptible to disease. This resulted in declining mortality rates and longer life spans. After centuries of fluctuations due to war, disease and famine, the total population of Europe started to increase beginning in 1750 (see McMahon 2006, p. 205).

The improvement of material conditions catalyzed by scientific advances was certainly an important factor contributing to the consolidation of the problematization of happiness in Western culture. After all, 'Only when individuals are free from the vicious daily pursuit of staying alive can they afford to undertake the pursuit of more exalted goals' in the present life (McMahon 2006, p. 205). Moreover, the evident material progress also further fueled the production of truth about pursuing the greatest amount of happiness for the greatest numbers.

Namely, inspired by the empirical investigations of natural laws and the concomitant technological progress, the Enlightenment thinkers also hoped to examine man and human laws with the same scientific precision.[11] Given the broad interest in happiness in the eighteenth century, it is not surprising that the new scientific approach based on mathematical gauges was quickly employed to examine and supposedly facilitate (public) happiness. If happiness has become the central goal of humanity, the Enlightenment thinkers believed, we should also attempt to measure the progress towards it. The Italian theorist Cesare Beccaria, for example, proposed

[11] Therefore, the Enlightenment thinkers are often considered to have made the first attempts of modern scientific analysis of man and society.

a 'political arithmetic' on which public policies towards 'greatest happiness shared among the greatest number' would be based and assessed (Beccaria 1986, p. 5). With the so-called Felicific calculus, Bentham (2000, Chap. 4) devised a more general approach with the help of which he hoped to be able to measure the degree or amount of pleasure that a specific action is likely to cause on both the individual and collective level. In another text, Bentham (1817) even tried to capture the play of pleasure and pain into a series of complex typologies that were supposed to define 'the springs of action' behind the principle of utility, which ranged from thirst and hunger to love and intoxication.

Perhaps the most notable attempt in this direction was Chastellux's historical comparative approach that begins in the typical Enlightenment spirit: 'are there any more beautiful, more worthy of our attention than those which have for their object the happiness of humanity? Many authors have examined with care, whether one people was more religious, more sober, or more warlike than another: none has yet attempted to find the happiest people' (Chastellux 1772 in Mcmahon 2006, p. 214). Aiming to fill these lacunae with what he called *indices de bonheur* (indicators of happiness), Chastellux's approach can be seen as one of the first empirical attempts to (comparatively) measure happiness. According to Chastellux, ideally this would require comparing variables such as daily and annual totals of working hours needed to acquire basic 'necessities and ease'; amount of available leisure time for the workers; levels of taxation, etc. Since such precise data was not available to him, he was, however, forced to adopt a more basic scale. Being well aware of the harsh material conditions of survival that plagued Europe for centuries (and which were now evidently improving), he saw the levels of population and the productivity of agriculture as the main positive indicators of public happiness. As for the negative ones, he regarded war and slavery as the main hindrances to public happiness, followed closely by religious superstition.

The next logical step of the emphasis on the advancement of knowledge about man and society was that rationally acquired knowledge should be employed for (moral) education and for determining the role the state and its government should play in the progress towards happiness.

For the Deists, happiness was ultimately a matter of conforming properly to the divine providential order intrinsically designed for the harmonic well-being of its inhabitants, but they were also less inclined to governmental and legislative intervention directly concerned with happiness. Of the many paths pursued by man, Locke (1993, p. 407) argued,

> There is only one of these which is the true way to eternal happiness. But in this great variety of ways that men follow, it is still doubted which is the right one. Now neither the care of the commonwealth, nor the right of enacting laws, does discover this way that leads to heaven more certainly to the magistrate, than every private man's search and study discovers it unto himself.

As a consequence, according to Locke, the matter of government was to enable individual liberty that would create the context in which citizens could pursue happiness on their own accord (by understanding the laws of the divine providential order): 'The great and chief end, therefore, of men's uniting into commonwealths and putting themselves under government,' Locke argues (2008, p. 76), 'is the preservation of their property' (where property for Locke corresponds both to material possessions and personal autonomy).

On the other hand, the Enlightenment philosophers refused the existence of divine providential order, and it followed that humans on their own ought to create a harmonic order that would—taking the natural causalities governing the play of pleasure and pain into account of course—enable the greatest happiness for the greatest number of people. A logical consequence of such rationale was that the Enlightenment philosophers were also more inclined to support a stronger role of government in ensuring happiness of its people.

Strongly believing in the idea of harmony of interests, the mainstream Enlightenment thinkers advocated progress towards individual and collective (public) happiness on the level of the state in both a positive sense—promoting happiness and eliminating suffering through education and the improvement of material conditions; and also in the negative sense of restraining the individual egoistic drive for pleasure through the laws and apparatuses of the state. In this sense, they saw important means for improvement of the human condition by way of education in relation to the government that would collectively provide the moral and political conditions for the happiness of society. Holbach, for example, argued that

> In fact, it is certain, that man is a social being, who in all things seeks his own happiness, that he does good when he finds it his interest; that he is not commonly bad, because that would be contrary to his welfare. This being premised let education teach men to know the relations which exist among themselves, and the arising from those relations; let governments calling to their aid laws, rewards and punishments, confirm the lessons given by education; let happiness accompany useful and virtuous actions, let shame, contempt, and chastisement be the rewards of vice. Then would mankind have a true morality, founded in their own nature upon their mutual and the interest of nations at large (Holbach 1761, Introduction).

Education, on the one hand, ought to cast away religious fanaticism and superstitions that, according to Enlightenment philosophers, prevented people pursuing earthly happiness as their true natural end. On the other hand, it should foster morality, wisdom and virtues in accordance with the idea of harmony of interest. 'Men,' in a typical paternalistic Enlightenment manor, Holbach emphasized (1995, p. 145), 'are only unhappy because they are ignorant'.

When referring to the state and government in relation to progress towards happiness, the majority of Enlightenment philosophers strongly emphasized that the state legislation and intervention should always follow the maxim of greatest happiness of its people: 'Every authority that is not exercised for the happiness of all can only be founded on imposture and force,' Chastellux insisted (in McMahon 2006, p. 217). In Benthams's (2000, Chap. 1) words, this implies that the principle of utility has to constitute the main principle 'not only of every action of a private individual,' but also of 'every measure of government':

> 'A measure of government which is but a particular kind of action, performed by a particular person or persons) may be said to be conformable to or dictated by the principle of utility, when in like manner the tendency which it has to augment the happiness of the community is greater than any which it has to diminish it' (Bentham 2000, Chap. 1).

In a similar vein, Adam Smith (2002, p. 216) also maintained that 'all constitutions of government… are valued only in proportion as they tend to promote the happiness of those who live under them. This is their sole use and end'.

According to the Enlightenment philosophers, the understanding of the state as serving and promoting the happiness of its inhabitants does not only mean that every state and its government has to always act in accordance with the maximization of happiness of its inhabitants, but also that such governance is in turn also serving the interest of the state itself. 'It is easy to convince every enlightened government,' Holbach argues (1761, Introduction),

> that it is their true interest to govern a happy people; that upon the happiness it procures the nation, depends the stability and safety of the government; in one word, that a nation composed of wise and virtuous citizens, are much more powerful than a troop of ignorant and corrupted slaves, whom the government is forced to deceive in order to satisfy, and to deluge with impositions that it may succeed in any enterprise.

Following from this, Holbach argues (1761, Chap. 16), let the rulers 'be careful to reward talents and virtue, to discourage inutility and punish vice, and their states will soon he filled with worthy and sensible citizens, who will feel it their own interest to serve and defend their country, and support the government which is the instrument of their felicity'. Interestingly enough, even though the majority of treatises concerning the role of the state come from European Enlightenment philosophers, happiness was institutionalized for the first time across the Atlantic with the famous lines of the American Declaration of Independence drafted by Thomas Jefferson in June, 1776: 'We hold these truths to be self-evident: that all men are created equal; that they are endowed by their creator with unalienable rights; that among these are life, liberty and the pursuit of happiness[12]'.

In regard to happiness in relation to the state, it is important to note that the treatises of Enlightenment philosophers concerning the role of the state and its government for the promotion of public happiness were mostly idealistic visions that were never entirely put into practice. As we shall see in the section analyzing the power axis constituting the modern experience of happiness, the actual political reality was quite different. Above we have argued that within the preceding experience of sin the vision of salvation was employed for the exercise of pastoral power. Similarly also within the modern experience of happiness the ideal of human existence was used for the exercise of (state) power. Namely, in practice, the idea of (public) happiness was strategically employed to primarily ensure, as Chemnitz (in Foucault 2007, p. 357) argued in as early as 1647, 'the state's preservation, expansion, and felicity' rather than the other way around as theoretically envisioned by the Enlightenment philosophers.

[12] Even though Jefferson's idea about the pursuit of happiness was largely inspired by European philosophers such as Locke and Hutcheson and although the early American settlers were mostly emigrants from Europe, the American experience of happiness had a specific development, which would require a particular examination that won't be pursued here.

Economic Progress and the Birth of Consumer Culture

In the beginning of the eighteenth century, *The Spectator*, one of the first influential daily publications in England, satirically portrayed two old-fashioned depictions of what could be called different strategies of human happiness of the time: on the one hand, the overzealous puritanism and, on the other, aristocratic libertinism. While the former were ridiculed as reactionary killjoys who still haven't grasped the open horizon of human progress promised by the Enlightenment, the latter were mocked for their excessive immoral debauchery. The progressive, pro-Enlightenment-oriented *The Spectator*, in contrast, advocated a middle path between the extremes, 'in which moderate pursuit of sober and rational pleasures would produce lasting enjoyment' (Porter 1996, p. 18). To that end, *The Spectator* 'stressed the importance of urbanity, politeness, rationality, moderation and the heeding of conventions, and gave fashionable sanction to the new sorts of pursuits—light reading, tea-table conversation, the pleasures of the town—expected to be personally gratifying while socially harmonious,' a view that was later imitated, recapitulated and further developed by numerous other writers and essayists.

The remaining reactionary forces, fearing that 'possessive individualism (pursuit of private gain) would prove to be disruptive' for society, were losing their momentum especially in the realm of the economy (Porter 1996, p. 17). The most explicit and most famous theoretical expression of the idea of harmony of interest in the economical field was Adam Smith's Wealth of Nations (1776/2007), which is widely considered to be the first modern economic theory. Amongst other things, Smith (1776/2007) argued that the selfish behavior of individuals as producers and consumers would result in the common good (provided that it is pursued in accordance with the competitive principles of the free market):

> Man has almost constant occasion for the help of his brethren, and it is in vain for him to expect it from their benevolence only./…/ It is not from the benevolence of the butcher, the brewer, or the baker, that we expect our dinner, but from their regard to their own interest. We address ourselves, not to their humanity but to their self-love, and never talk to them of our own necessities but of their advantages. Nobody but a beggar chooses to depend chiefly upon the benevolence of his fellow-citizens (Smith 2007, p. 9).

In practice, liberal economic doctrine pioneered by Smith (1776/2007) was starting to be increasingly employed only in the nineteenth century. The actual economic growth, however, was well under way already under the reign of mercantilism, the preceding economic doctrine dominating Europe from the sixteenth to the eighteenth century. In accordance with the political rationality of the time (which will be examined in more detail in the section about power), mercantilism can be seen as an early form of capitalism that advocated the economic growth of the state through state-oriented protectionism.

Nascent industrialization and increasing economic growth, international trade and the expansion of urban centers on the one side produced new concentrated markets and an increased supply and variety of consumer goods. On the other, they resulted in 'a more commercial, money-driven capitalist economy, which left more people with spare money in their pockets to be spent or squandered on a growing range of amusements and commodities' (Porter 1996, p. 19). These processes catalyzed what historians call the birth of consumer culture/society (McKendrick et al. 1985; Roche 2000), which enabled new and increasing forms of sensual enjoyments hitherto reserved for aristocratic elites to start becoming accessible to a wider array of people and eventually to the masses[13]. In turn, 'enlightened economists and progressive social commentators began to view culture, sport and leisure as productive and valuable sectors of the economy, as forces of civilization and social cohesion, and as indices of improvement' (Porter 1996, p. 23). In this context, besides the industry producing commodities, a new kind of industry also arose, devoted exclusively to satisfying the popular thirst for pleasures' (Porter 1996, p. 23). For the first time, Porter further explains (1996, p. 23), 'There emerged sizable bodies of professional actors, theatre managers, painters, sportsmen, art dealers, journalists, hack writers, and other people whose business was to provide entertainment for the public at large'.

The birth of a consumer culture that enables and facilitates the Enlightenment pursuit of sensual pleasure should, therefore, be seen as closely connected to the birth of happiness. Or, as the French economist and statesman Jaques Turgot, known for making the first explicit statement on progress (1750), vividly observed, the people of his time 'as it were, bought and sold happiness' (Turgot in Rothschild 2001, p. 242).

Idealizing the idea of progress at all levels of human society, the prospects for improving the human condition on earth for many Enlightenment philosophers seemed virtually endless. Bentham, for example (1983, I.4), observed that 'in civilized nations, and therefore in the whole of mankind, the sum of well-being is perpetually on the increase'. In this sense, he (and also Voltaire, 1764) regarded the scholastic and classical belief in the highest good (Summum Bonum) as a final place of rest merely as a misguided search for a 'philosopher's stone' that was 'meaningless and absurd'. 'The desire for bettering our condition,' the eighteenth-century social commentator Frederick Eden insisted (in Porter 1996, p. 12), 'is the predominant principle that animates the world'. And, according to the principle of utility, pleasure could always be further increased and suffering could always be further reduced.

Even though the Enlightenment vision of happiness through progress is explicitly constituted in direct contrast to the preceding Christian experience of sin, it paradoxically retained certain latent sediments of its logic. Akin to the idea of salvation, the vision of progress towards happiness is also based on firm and clear foundations. The certainty of God's wisdom, laws and mercy is replaced by deep faith in the power of reason believed to enable insight into the ultimate truth about achieving happiness in the present life.

In contrast to the Christian ideal of existence understood as a possible future prospect in the life to come, the Enlightenment promised that happiness could be rightly pursued and is attainable already (and only) in this life. However—and this

[13] In spite of the general growth of affluence resulting in a more inclusive consumer culture, there were still considerable class class-related differences in consumption patterns.

is the paradox—the promise of happiness through progress only exists as an ideal in the horizon of the future, a condition indeed achievable on Earth, but still not quite yet achieved. In this sense, 'the promised land in the future,' envisioned by the Enlightenment idea of progress towards happiness, Bruckner argues (2010, p. 32),

> recedes before us and strangely resembles the Christian beyond. It evaporates every time we try to seize it, disappoints us as soon as we approach it. Whence the ambiguities of the idea of progress: it is a call for effort, courage, and the hope of succeeding where earlier generations failed, but it is also a defense of present suffering in the name of an improvement postponed to an enchanting but distant future. "Tomorrow" once again becomes the eternal category of sacrifice, and historical optimism takes on the appearance of an endless purgation. Eden will always come later on.

In addition, the traces of Christian logic in the Enlightenment vision of happiness can be also found in the idea of harmony of interest and public happiness. The mainstream Enlightenment movement indeed clearly connects happiness to the pursuit of sensual pleasures. However, the idea of harmony of interest behind the ideal of public happiness still implies a certain restraint of the inherent human desire for maximizing pleasure and minimizing pain. While within the Christian experience of sin the desire had to be restrained in the name of God and salvation, now it has to be restrained (to a much lesser extent, though) in the name of reason and for public happiness.

In order to further explore the process of birth of happiness, let us now turn to the axis of ethics and look more closely to the relationship to the self constituting the experience of happiness.

The Modern Subject of Happiness

Above, we have argued that in the Christian experience of salvation, *the telos* was about achieving purity (of desire), which was supposed to lead to salvation and true bliss in heaven. Already in the seventeenth century, we can see that the telos started to transform and change its focus. According to the more rational Christianity developing at the time culminating in the Deist philosophy, it would be unkind in the extreme for God to create humans that would suffer through no fault of their own and without giving them the capacities to determine how to act rightly to merit happiness both in this world and in the life to come. Questioning original sin, emphasizing rationality and reaffirming pleasure, Deism and the accompanying wider social and religious developments, thus, restored the capacities of human beings to achieve the ideal of human existence in this world.

While within the Christian problematization of salvation human desire for pleasure had to be neutralized because it leads to sin and uncleanliness, now earthly pleasure and happiness are put to the fore. Although the prospect of afterlife is still there, the cardinal telos towards the end of the seventeenth century increasingly became happiness and pleasure on earth. The reference to God and heaven is, therefore, not 'wholly absent, but it seems to be subordinate to a conception of happiness which is defined purely in creaturely terms' (Taylor 2001, p. 267). Already in his early years, Locke wrote the following lines in his journal: 'The business of man… [is] to be happy in this world by enjoyment of the things of nature subservient to life health ease and pleasure and the comfortable hopes of another life when this is ended' (Locke in Wilson 2007, p. 401). According to the Deist view, this is possible because 'God is kind enough to make our acting for our present happiness the way of securing our future goods; which is to say that the rewards and punishments of a future life endorse the path which produces the most mutual happiness in this' (Tindal in Taylor 2001, p. 245). In this sense, 'happiness is the attaining of the things we by nature desire, or pleasure in the absence of pain' and 'the rewards of the next life seem to be considered just as more intense and longer-lasting versions of the pleasures and pains of this' (Taylor 2001, p. 267).

Telos in the secular experience of happiness brought by the Enlightenment is a logical derivate of the Deist telos. Based on the intensification of problematization of positive feeling/pleasure and the affirmation of everyday life, the Enlightenment vision of happiness is characterized by "the modern naturalist-utilitarian hostility to 'higher' goods and defense of ordinary, sensuous happiness" (Taylor 2001, p. 104). It, hence, further emphasizes happiness, pleasure and sensual fulfillment as the ultimate human goal, but understands it exclusively in earthly terms: 'Let man cease to search outside of the world he lives in, for beings that provide him with a happiness which nature refuses him' (Holbach 1966, p. 3). Following from this, du Chatelet argues (in McMahon 2006, p. 210), 'there is nothing more to do in this life than to procure for ourselves agreeable sentiments and sensations'. For some Enlightenment writers, happiness was not only considered a universal human possibility, but almost an imperative. In 1738, for example, the young Mirabeau wrote a letter to his friend Vauvenargues criticizing him for not having an explicit strategy of happiness: 'See here, my friend, you think all the time, you study, and nothing is beyond the scope of your ideas; and yet you never think for a moment about making a clear plan leading to what should be our only goal: happiness' (Mirabeau in Bruckner 2010, p. 1). In sum, Porter explains (1996, p. 3), what therefore

> marks the innovativeness of the eighteenth century is its new accent upon the legitimacy of pleasure—not as occasional release, aristocratic paganism or heavenly bliss, but as the routine entitlement of people at large to seek fulfillment in this world rather than only in heavenly salvation, to achieve the gratification of the senses not just the purification of the soul. (Porter 1996, p. 3)

Still partly adhering to the Christian tradition, the mode of subjection in the religious experience of happiness is the Law of God also designated by some authors as the law of nature, law of reason or natural justice. Regardless of the differences in nomenclature, Deists agreed that this universal principle is based on divine providential order inherently designed by the creator for the common good and happiness of its inhabitants. According to Adam Smith, for example (2002, p. 279),

> the administration of the great system of the universe, however, the care of the universal happiness of all rational and sensible beings, is the business of God and not of man. To man is allotted a much humbler department, but one much more suitable to the weakness of his powers, and to the narrowness of his comprehension; the care of his own happiness, of that of his family, his friends, his country.

Compared to the medieval Christian notion of a hierarchical universe manifested in the ladder of being, or to the Protestant idea of predestination according to which only the few chosen ones can be saved, the Deist notion of providential order and God's law is much less severe and more inclusive. Namely, according to this new rational Christianity, God is kind enough to make a law according to which human pursuit for the present happiness and pleasure is at the same time also the best way of securing future well-being. As for the details of God's law for us, Tindal explains, a Deist philosopher who pushed Locke's arguments to their logical conclusion, "We only have to look into the 'Book of Nature' to see what relations we stand in, and what they require[14]. Only a tyrant would impose commands which do not flow from these relations" (Tindal in Taylor 2001, p. 245).

Above, we have argued that the religious experience of happiness differs from the Christian experience of sin in almost all major facets. The only aspect in which it maintains a certain continuity with the Christian experience of sin is its mode of subjection, which is still founded on divine law. As a consequence, this is also the aspect most fundamentally transformed by the Enlightenment process of secularization, which has replaced the law of God based on God's providential design with nature and its contingent causal relations. After abandoning God as the foundation of happiness, Holbach argues (1966, p. 2), let man 'study nature, that he learn its laws, that he contemplate its energy and the immutable way it acts; let him apply his discoveries to his own felicity, and submit in silence to laws from whose binding force nothing can remove him'.

Holbach's (1966) *Systeme de la nature* was one of the first systematic and uncompromising expressions of the shift from rational Christianity to naturalism and materialism. According to this view, human individuals, like everything else in the universe, are entirely physical. Undercutting the divine foundation of human morality and happiness, materialism sees the moral dimension in man simply in terms of his physical existence considered 'from a certain point of view, that is relative to some of his ways of acting' (Holbach 1966, p. 3). Inspired by the growing natural sciences and Spinozist monism, (Holbach's) materialism also means that physics can offer us an understanding of human existence by revealing analogies between the natural processes on all levels of existence:

> Self-preservation is thus the common goal towards which all energies, forces, and human faculties seem continuously directed. Scientists have named this tendency or direction gravitation to a centre. Newton calls it force of inertia, moralists have called it in man self-love, which is but the tendency to preserve oneself, the desire for happiness, the love of well-being and pleasure ... This gravitation is thus a necessary disposition in man and all beings, who, by diverse means, tend to persevere in the existence they have received, as long as nothing disturbs the order of their machine or its primitive tendency. (Holbach 1966, p. 58)

The Enlightenment vision of man driven by the necessity to self-preservation and the inclination to maximize pleasure is understood 'not just as the correct conclu-

[14] While a similar observation pertaining to natural laws was made much earlier by Galileo Galilei, the Deist innovation was that from the "Book of Nature" it is also possible to draw inductive conclusions about ethical and soteriological questions.

sion of observing reason but also as the deliverance of ultimately undistorted moral insight' (Taylor 2001, p. 326). The Enlightenment, therefore, 'embraced materialism and atheism not just as the ultimate deliverance of self-responsible reason but also as the way of being integrally true to the demand of nature' (Taylor 2001, p. 325). This, along with the understanding of nature as the mode of subjection, is clearly exposed in Bentham, who argued that 'nature has placed mankind under the governance of two sovereign masters, pain and pleasure. It is for them alone to point out what we ought to do, as well as to determine what we shall do. On the one hand, the standard of right and wrong, on the other the chain of causes and effects, are fastened to their throne' (Bentham 2000, Chap. 1).

The ethical substance within the Christian experience of sin was desire and concupiscence for the pleasures of the flesh, which had to be neutralized in order to reach the telos—purity. Refusing such demands for the transcendence of nature by endorsing the fulfillments of ordinary life, already Deism and the accompanying wider social developments have initiated a fundamental transformation of ethical substance. The Enlightenment has taken this transformation towards the problematization of (good) feeling and sentiment another step further. First, Taylor explains (2001, p. 327), 'if Deism had defended the innocence of ordinary human desire from the hyper-Augustinian charge of thoroughgoing perversion through sin, this could be done all the more effectively in completely rejecting the religion within which the notion of sin took its sense'. And second, 'if Deism had defended the value of ordinary life against the supposedly higher goals of traditional ethics, naturalism could do this all the more uncompromisingly by stressing the centrality of physical pleasure and fulfillment' (Taylor 2001, p. 327).

In this sense, both the religious and the secular experiences of happiness radically overturned the preceding Christian formula of neutralizing desire for the pleasures of the flesh, already eroded to a certain extent by humanism and reformation through the problematization of (good) feeling. Now—on the contrary—desire has to be fulfilled because it alone can lead to achieving telos, which has now become earthly pleasure in the form of happiness. On account of this, Diderot, the famous father of the encyclopedia, remarked, 'I don't know what this thing is you call religion, but I can only think badly of it, since it prevents you from tasting an innocent pleasure, to which nature, the sovereign mistress, invites us all' (Diderot in Taylor 2001, p. 329). It is revealing that Bentham (in Taylor 2001, p. 328) also saw the 'principle of asceticism' as the cardinal antipode of the principle of utility.

Following from this in the Enlightenment period, 'the promotion of ordinary life, already transposed by Deists into an affirmation of the pursuit of happiness begins to turn into an exaltation of the sensual' (Taylor 2001, p. 328). Ethical substance, therefore, becomes constituted by feeling and the sensual.

Practices of Pleasure and Happiness

In line with the aspects of the relationship to the self and the transformations of the other axis of experience, the birth of happiness affirmed and gave rise to a plethora of practices of pleasure, which are—according to the principle of utility—supposed to bring happiness to individuals: 'as uncertainty grew about the prospect of a heavenly reward,' Thomas explains (2009, p. 266), 'most people, without explicitly declaring any religious skepticism, chose in practice to devote their main energies to the business of making this life as fulfilling as possible'.

In direct contrast to the preceding Christian asceticism and the glorification of suffering, people of the Enlightenment sought pleasures in a variety of new forms, many of which were invented and provided in the context of the developing consumer culture. As we have argued above, this developing consumer culture also enabled a much wider array of people to participate in buying commodities. On the one side, we, therefore, have an increased demand for various practices of pleasure, and on the other, 'the market—or in other words commercial opportunism—that led the way in providing new forms of entertainment for the paying crowd[15]' (Porter 1996, p. 32).

The developing consumer practices were 'accompanied and facilitated by new marketing and advertising techniques' (Thomas 2009, p. 119). The increased variety, quality and quantity of the stock coming from rapidly developing industrialization and international trade were followed by 'improvements in methods of sale and distribution, reflected in the increasing separation of retailing from production, a rise in the number of shops, chapmen, and other outlets' (Thomas 2009, p. 119). While these developments could more or less be observed across Europe, England with its large empire and the most rapidly developing level of industrialization was leading the way in consumer revolution. 'It is almost impossible to express how well everything is organized in London,' the German novelist, Sophie von La Roche (1933), admired in 1786:

> Every article is made more attractive to the eye than in Paris or any other town. We especially noticed a cunning device for showing women's materials Whether they are silks, chintzes or muslins, they hang down in folds behind the fine high windows so that the effect of this or that material, as it would be in the ordinary folds of a woman's dress can be studied. Amongst the muslins all colors are on view, and so one can judge how the frock would like in company with its fellows. Now large shoe and slipper shops for anything from adults down to dolls can be seen—now fashion articles or silver or brass shops—boots, guns, glasses—the confectioner's goodies, the pewterer's wares—fans, etc. Behind great glass windows absolutely everything one can think of is neatly, attractively displayed, and in such abundance of choice as almost to make one greedy.

Besides buying happiness by refining their personal style, early modern consumers also sought pleasure in improving the appearance and comfort of their homes that were "increasingly stocked with comforts and 'decencies,' which were shop-bought rather than home-made' even in ordinary people's homes: from 'curtains to carpets, tableware to tea-sets, plate to prints' (Porter 1996, p. 23).

---

[15] Within the preceding experience of sin, a lot of attention and ingenuity was dedicated to designing objects that produced suffering (as we have seen above, there was a strong competition between the craftsmen of torture instruments, which even had "catchy" names that, to a certain extent, resemble consumer brands). Within the modern experience of happiness, the competing efforts in the context of emerging capitalism are now directed to produce various objects of pleasure.

Shopping as the cardinal consumer practice, therefore, started acquiring new functions: from a practice of procuring basic needs of survival, it developed into a leisure activity[16]. In this sense, Thomas explains (2009, p. 121), "many of the goods purchased in the early modern period were acquired, not for convenience or to satisfy a physical need, but to allay what many commentators were learning to call 'imaginary,' 'artificial,' or 'phantastic' wants".

The consumer culture also included a variety of new (such as leisure reading of books, essays, novels, light reading and magazines) and the intensification of old kinds of amusements such as food and drink. As Porter (1996, p. 33) observes, 'enormous delight was taken in food—partly as a result of low prices, partly thanks to the increasing importation of new and exotic foodstuffs such as pineapples'. Culinary indulgences were then washed down by those of the bottle. The eighteenth century especially 'was notorious for heavy alcohol consumption, indeed for public and often unashamed drunkenness' (Porter 1996, p. 33), which was becoming all the more intensive as it was precisely in this time that the much stronger distilled spirits 'became available' and gained 'widespread popularity throughout Europe' (Martin 2001, p. 18).

What we therefore see 'during the seventeenth and eighteenth centuries,' Thomas explains (2009, p. 140)

> is the gradual emergence of a new ideology, accepting the pursuit of con- summer goods as a valid object of human endeavor, and recognizing that no limit could, or should, be put to it. Consumption was justified in terms of the opportunities it brought for human fulfillment. The growth of a consumer market, unrestricted by the requirements of social hierarchy, offered increasing possibilities for comfort, enjoyment, and self-realization. Poverty was no longer to be regarded as a holy state; and there was no need to feel guilt about envying the rich; one should try to emulate them.

Sport was also influenced and transformed by the Enlightenment call for pleasure. While hitherto it was mostly practiced as 'part of ritual activity,' in the eighteenth century sport was 'developed on professional and commercial lines encouraging the emergence of the paying spectator' (Porter 1996, p. 30); and, of course, people also exercised in their beds. Indulgence in sexual activities—considered in the preceding Christian experience of sin as the source of the gravest sins—was becoming more accepted as the legitimate practice of pleasure. According to Porter (1996, p. 34), recent scholarship has shown evidence indicating that in the eighteenth century (in England at least) 'sex was publicly flaunted' in a 'manor that bears comparison with the second half of the twentieth century'[17]. Judging this trend by the rate of prosti-

[16] While the increase in consumerism as a pleasurable practice or as a leisure activity was no longer only reserved for the elites, it remained an 'expression to the social hierarchy' (Thomas 2009, p. 118). In this sense, Thomas explains (2009, p. 118), 'possessions were used to signify power, wealth, ancestry, mental cultivation, and nobility of character. As a result, most commodities acquired a distinctive set of symbolic meanings and associations, full of social resonance. To possess them was inevitably an act of self-definition'.

[17] For a more thorough reflection of this theme one should also consider Foucault's analysis of the modern sexuality in the History of Sexuality Vol. 1 (1978) that attempts to illuminate how

tution, it is revealing that at the time in London alone, 'there were anything up to 30,000 public streetwalkers' (Porter 1996, p. 34).

Publicly, new consumer and amusement practices were most intensively pursued in the cities. In this sense, the city was increasingly becoming 'a social and cultural centre, designed for the spending of surplus money on enjoyments and entertainments' (Porter 1996, p. 25). Besides the already mentioned shops in many cities, special venues and institutions 'devoted to pleasure-taking' were springing up: 'assembly rooms, theaters and halls for meetings and performances, with space set aside for clubs, lectures, spectacles, displays and other events' (Porter 1996, p. 26). Probably the best example of a locus reserved for practices of pleasure are the so-called pleasures gardens such as Vauxhall and Ranelagh Gardens in England and in Paris at the Palais Royal. Pleasure gardens were a kind of proto-amusement park established for the purpose of pleasure and enjoyment, 'offering games and recreation, spectacles and refreshments, music, and sanctuaries in which lovers could stroll' (McMahon 2006, p. 199).

Certain towns (such as Bath, Buxton and Scarborough in England) were even chiefly devoted to offering a variety of practices of pleasure that were often also accompanied with the facilities for recovery and health. These "pleasure resort towns" 'specialized in pump rooms and assembly rooms where tea could be taken, balls held, and gambling indulged—to say nothing of amorous assignations,' Porter explains (1996, p. 27). It is certainly revealing that the notorious conservative theologian Charles Wesley, who was one of the founders of Methodism,[18] described Bath as 'hell on earth' (Wesley in Porter 1996, p. 27).

Insofar as the emphasis on pleasure constitutes the central element of the modern experience of happiness, Porter's (1996, p. 1) observation 'that pleasure came into its own in the eighteenth century' supports our thesis about the birth of happiness in the seventeenth and especially eighteenth century. After centuries of Christian suppression of the sensual, the goal of an increasing number of people became to enjoy themselves, to pursue happiness through pleasure and to have fun. It is revealing (and at the same time also supportive of our thesis about the birth of happiness in the seventeenth and the eighteenth centuries) that semantically the word fun 'was a relative novelty, introduced in English only in the late seventeenth century as a variation of the Middle English *fon*, meaning jester or fool' (McMahon 2006, p. 199).

Last but not least, it is important to add that even though the developing consumer culture enabled a much wider array of people to participate in different practices of pleasure described above, economic circumstances still 'limited the ability of many to take advantage of the new freedom' (Thomas 2009, p. 140). Towards the end of the seventeenth century, for example, Thomas observes (2009, p. 140), 'a quarter of the population endured some form of poverty and a seventh were in or near destitution'.

---

sex towards the end of the eighteenth and in the nineteenth century has been 'put into discourse' (Foucault 1978, p. 11).

[18] Methodism was an evangelical movement that emerged in the eighteenth century in the United Kingdom.

In the next section that will focus on the relation between happiness and the state in the context of relations of power, we shall see that not all the practices and techniques constituting the early modern experience of happiness served the pursuit of individual pleasures.

Modern Experience of Happiness and Power

Above, we have seen that with pastoral power constituting an important part of the Christian experience of sin in the Middle Ages, the Christian Church introduced a new unique form of power to Western culture that was individualizing, totalizing and salvation-oriented. In spite of the fact that this pastoral power—as we have also argued—was even further reinforced by the outcomes of pastoral struggles during the Reformation and counter-Reformation, one might suppose that the secularization processes and the replacement of the problematization of salvation with the problematization of happiness induced in the Enlightenment period resulted in its disappearance or at least in the loss of the main part of its efficacy. Foucault (2002, p. 333) warns, however, that one has to be careful with such a simple generalization because 'we should distinguish two aspects of pastoral power—between the ecclesiastical institutionalization that has created or at least lost its vitality since the eighteenth century, and its function, which has spread and multiplied outside the ecclesiastical institution'.

We shall argue that the spread and the multiplication of pastoral modality of power outside the Church institution that eventually resulted in 'the state as a modern matrix of individualization' (Foucault 2002, p. 334) is largely also connected to the process of the birth of the modern experience of happiness in the seventeenth and the eighteenth centuries. More precisely, in this chapter, we shall examine the new political rationality called raison d'etat (reason of state) and its political technology, the police[19], which, in the seventeenth and eighteenth centuries, sprouted on the substrate of pastoral power and which constituted the power axis of the early modern experience of happiness. Similarly, as within the preceding experience of sin, where the vision of salvation was primarily employed to reinforce the mechanisms of pastoral power, also within the modern experience of happiness the idea of (public) happiness—the successor of the idea of salvation—was strategically employed to guide political technologies used to increase the strength or happiness of the state.

[19] As we shall see, the understanding of police in the early modern period was quite different and much broader than it is now.

Raison of the State and the Birth of Modern Experience of Happiness

Above, we have seen how the rationalism represented one of the currents resulting in the birth of happiness on the axis of truth. Starting with the natural theologians and the Deists, and then culminating in the Enlightenment movement, reason became the cardinal foundation of human progress towards happiness. In this sense, rationality was perceived as something inherently good and unproblematic that is in direct contrast to the irrational (which, for the Enlightenment thinkers, was mostly embodied in the preceding Christian experience).

Firstly, because he thinks "it's senseless to refer to 'reason' as the contrary entity to non-reason[20]" and, secondly, because every rationalization is always linked to relations of power, Foucault (2002, p. 299) is extremely critical towards such an unreflexive glorification of rationality, which in his view should rather be perceived as a potentially 'dangerous' concept. Following from this, Foucault (2002, p. 299) further argues, 'the main problem when people try to rationalize something is not to investigate whether or not they conform to principles of rationality but to discover which kind of rationality they are using'. What we therefore have to do 'is analyze specific rationalities rather than always invoking the progress of rationalization in general' (Foucault 2002, p. 329).

In this spirit, we shall investigate the political reason called reason of state (*raison d'etat*) and its main political technology, the police, which constituted the power axis of the (early) modern experience of happiness in the seventeenth and eighteenth centuries. According to Foucault (2002, p. 417), political rationality is always

> linked with other forms of rationality. Its development in large part is dependent upon economical, social, cultural, and technical processes. It is always embodied in institutions' strategies and has its own specificity. Since political rationality is the root of a great number of postulates, commonplaces of all sorts, institutions and ideas we take for granted, it is both theoretically and practically important to go on with this historical criticism, this historical analysis of our political rationality, which is something different from the discussion about political theories and which is different also from divergences between different political choices.

First, let us look more closely at the main development that brought about the transition from the pastoral government of souls based on the problematization of salvation to the political government of men and populations based on the problematization of happiness. In order to understand how the pastoral individualizing form of government transformed and spread outside of the Church institution, we first have to return to Aquinas who explains the nature of the royal power characteristic of the medieval experience of sin.

According to Foucault (2007, p. 309), in Aquinas's understanding of the king, 'there is no discontinuity, no specificity, and no division between the two functions

[20] Foucault (2002, p. 299) further explains that 'such trail would trap us into playing the arbitrary and boring part of either the rationalist or the irrationalist'.

of being sovereign and governing'. Namely, Aquinas defines the type of the government ensured by the monarch, the sovereign with the help of three models.

As Foucault explains, for Aquinas, 'the king's art will be excellent insofar as it imitates nature, that is to say insofar as it operates like God. And just as God created nature, the king will be the founder of the state or city, and just as God governs nature, the king will govern his state, city, or province'. The first model is hence based on the analogy with God. The second analogy is with nature itself. According to Aquinas, 'the body of a man and of any other animal would fall apart if there were not some general ruling force to sustain the body and secure the common good of all its parts' (Aquinas in Foucault 2007, p. 310). Insofar as Aquinas's logic applies to the kingdom, Foucault explains (2007, p. 310), 'there must be something in the kingdom that corresponds to the vital, guiding force in the organism, and this is the king, who turns each individual's tendency back from his own good towards the common good'. And the third analogy is with the pastor and the *pater familias*. Above, we have seen that for Aquinas the ultimate goal of man is eternal bliss found in the enjoyment of God and following from this is also the royal function: 'because the end of our living well at this present time is the blessedness of heaven,' Aquinas argues, 'the king's duty is therefore to secure the good life for the community [*multitudo*] in such a way as to ensure that it is led to the blessedness of heaven' (Aquinas in Foucault 2007, p. 310).

Governing in accordance with these three models ensures that there is no break in the great continuum of sovereignty extending from God to the monarch (and then further down to the father of the family). Through this continuum, God governs the world in a pastoral sense, which, according to Foucault (2007, p. 312), means that

> the things of the world were made for man and that man was not made to live in this world, at any rate not definitively, but only in order to pass into another world. The world governed in a pastoral fashion according to a system of salvation was [therefore] a world of final causes that culminated in man who had to earn his salvation in this world. Final causes and anthropocentrism was one of the forms, one of the manifestations, one of the signs of God's pastoral government of the world.

The second characteristic of pastoral government of the world was 'that the world was subject to a system of obedience,' which effectively meant that God actively intervened in the world and 'forced beings to show his will through signs, prodigies, marvels, and monstrosities that were so many threats of chastisement, promises of salvation, or marks of election' (Foucault 2007, p. 311). Finally, the world subject to the pastoral government of God 'was a world in which there was an entire system of truth: truth taught, on the one hand, and truth hidden and extracted on the other' (Foucault 2007, p. 311).

Towards the end of the sixteenth and in the beginning of the seventeenth century, the concept of pastoral governance of the world was challenged by developing scientific practices, which we have already mentioned above on the truth axis and which included empirical approaches such as natural theology (John Ray), physics (Galileo), astronomy (Copernicus, Kepler), Port Royal Grammar, etc.[21] Namely, the

---

[21] These developments of knowledge coincide with the foundation of 'the classical episteme,' which Foucault describes in The Order of Things (2005).

new empiricist perspective implied that God does not govern the world in the pastoral sense, but 'in a sovereign manner through principles' (Foucault 2007, p. 311); that is, 'through general, immutable, and universal laws, through simple and intelligible laws that are accessible either in the form of measurement and mathematical analysis, or in the form of classificatory analysis in the case of natural history[22] (Foucault 2007, p. 311). The conception of nature based on the new scientific approach 'no longer tolerates government' and 'only allows the reign of a reason that is ultimately the common reason of God and men' (Foucault 2007, p. 313). While before nature was marked by constant divine governance and intervention, now 'nature only allows a reason that has fixed once and for all' general laws or principles of nature [*principia naturae*] (Foucault 2007, p. 313).

The erosion of God's pastoral governance of the world (or as Foucault also calls this process—the 'de-governmentalization of the cosmos') towards the end of the sixteenth century resulted in breaking the uninterrupted continuum of sovereignty 'which justifies the king's government of men' (Foucault 2007, p. 311). Of course, this does not mean that 'the relationship of the sovereign, or of a person who governs, to God, to nature, to the father of a family, and to the religious pastor is broken' (Foucault 2007, p. 311). Rather, it corresponds to a need for a new kind of problematization of sovereignty marked by 'the pursuit and definition of a specific form of government with respect to the exercise of sovereignty' (Foucault 2007, p. 311).

Insofar, according to the new conception of God's governance of the world, as 'the sovereign's exercise of sovereignty over his subjects is not distinguished simply by his extension of divine sovereignty over Earth that would somehow be reflected in the continuum of nature,' the sovereign has to perform a specific task of governing, the model for which is 'found neither in God nor in nature' (Foucault 2007, p. 313). 'In relation to his sovereignty, and in relation to the pastorate,' Foucault explains (2007, p. 313), 'something more is demanded from him, something different, something else. This is government'.

On the one hand, we therefore have the universal principle governing the natural world and, on the other, we have a 'sovereignty over men that is required to take upon itself something specific that is not directly contained in it, which conforms to another model and another type of rationality'[23] (Foucault 2007, p. 313). And insofar as this new kind of problematization cannot rely on existing models, it has to find a new model, a new political rationality 'in accordance with which we will be able to carry out this operation' (Foucault 2007, p. 313). This new model of art of government that emerged towards the end of the sixteenth century is ratio status—raison d'Etat—reason of state[24].

---

[22] These developments have eventually resulted in the understanding of the world as the divine providential order designed by God for the well-being of its inhabitants adopted by the Deists (see above).

[23] According to Foucault (2007, p. 314), 'with principia naturae and ratio status, principles of nature and raison d'État, nature and state, the two great references of the knowledge (savoirs) and techniques given to modern Western man are finally constituted, or finally separated'.

[24] Being based on the refusal of the old Christian understanding of the cosmos it is hardly surprising that some orthodox Christian thinkers assimilated the political theory of reason of state to atheism.

The first definitions of reason of state were provided by Botero, Palazzo (Discourse on Government and True Reason of State 1606) and Chemnitz (De Ratione status 1647). According to Foucault (2002, p. 314), all these definitions share the following characterizations of reason of state. First, "reason of state is regarded as an 'art,' that is, a technique conforming to certain rules," which 'do not simply pertain to customs or traditions,' but (in line with the emphasis on rational enquiry in this period) 'to knowledge—rational knowledge' (Foucault 2002, p. 314).

Second, reason of state is positioned in stark contrast to the Machiavellian tradition, which was an important and controversial issue in the literature on government in this period. In "The Prince," Foucault explains (2002, p. 407), 'Machiavelli's problem is to decide how a province or a territory acquired through inheritance or conquest can be held against internal and external rivals'. As a consequence, 'Machiavelli's entire analysis is aimed at defining what keeps up or reinforces the link between prince and the state' (Foucault 2002, p. 407). The theoreticians of reason of state, on the other hand, are interested in 'the very existence and nature of this new entity which is the state itself' (Foucault 2002, p. 407). The theoreticians of reason of state, therefore, refused Machiavelli not only because in this period he had a very bad reputation, but primarily because 'they couldn't recognize their own problem in his problem' (Foucault 2002, p. 407). According to Foucault (2002, p. 407), reason of state, therefore, introduced an innovation in political rationality that was fundamentally different from that of Machiavelli: 'the aim of this new art of governing is precisely not to reinforce the power of the prince. Its aim is to reinforce state itself' (Foucault 2002, p. 407).

An important consequence of this new political rationality was that the project of reconstituting the Roman Empire, which was based on the widely accepted medieval idea 'that all the kingdoms of the earth would be one day unified in one last empire just before Christ's return to earth,' completely disappears from the political thought (Foucault 2002, p. 408). Insofar as 'the state only exists through and for itself, and it only exists in the plural' (Foucault 2008, p. 5), 'politics has now to deal with an irreducible multiplicity of states struggling and competing' between each other (Foucault 2002, p. 409).

Finally, insofar as reason of state is perceived as rational government aimed at increasing the strength of the state in comparison to other competing states, it also presupposes the need for knowledge about the state's capacities, the means to enlarge it and the capacities of other states (Foucault 2002, p. 316). Such specialized knowledge not only entails 'implementing general principles of reason, wisdom, and prudence,' but 'concrete, precise, and measured knowledge as to the state's strength' (Foucault 2002, p. 316). Following from this political rationality of reason of state was "intimately bound up with the development of what was then called either political 'statistics' or 'arithmetic'; that is, the knowledge of different states' respective forces" (Foucault 2002, p. 317)[25].

[25] Above in the section about progress towards happiness we have already mentioned several examples of such knowledge.

In sum, the new political rationality called reason of state that emerged towards the end of the sixteenth and in the beginning of the seventeenth century 'defined the state and separated it out as both a specific and an autonomous, or relatively autonomous, reality' (Foucault 2008, p. 4). The government of the state must still 'respect divine, moral, and natural laws as laws which are not homogeneous with or intrinsic to the state' (Foucault 2008, p. 4). However, while 'in the Middle Ages the sovereign was commonly defined as someone who must help his subjects gain their salvation in the next world,' the government now 'has to do something other than ensure the salvation of its subjects in the hereafter' (Foucault 2008, p. 4). In line with the transformations induced in the process of the birth of happiness on the axis of truth and relation to the self, the goal of government according to reason of the state now becomes ensuring happiness.

Above, we have seen that, even though royal government 'did indeed fall under a particular terrestrial art,' its final objective within the experience of sin was to 'ensure that on leaving their terrestrial status, and freed from this human republic, men can arrive at eternal bliss and the enjoyment of God' (Foucault 2007, p. 340). The reason of state fundamentally changed the end around which this—also called *res publica*—had to be organized. According to reason of state, 'there is no prior, external purpose, or even a purpose subsequent to the state itself' (Foucault 2007, p. 340). The new end, the new problematization of res publica was now 'the state itself and if there is something like perfection, happiness, or felicity, it will only ever be the perfection, happiness, or felicity of the state itself' (Foucault 2007, p. 340). Chemnitz (1647 in Foucault 2007, p. 357), for example, defines the reason of state as 'a certain political consideration required for all public matters, councils and projects, whose only aim is the state's preservation, expansion, and felicity; to which end, the easiest and promptest means are to be employed'.

Chimnitz's definition points to the fact that the early conceptions of reason of state explicitly referred to happiness of the state and not to happiness of individuals or the population of this state. In this sense, Foucault explains (2007, p. 357), 'it is not men who must be happy or prosperous, and ultimately it is not men who must be rich; it is the state itself[26]'.

The inability of the early theoreticians of reason of state to conceive of happiness in terms of the state's population was connected to the fact that 'population had not yet entered into the reflexive prism' (Foucault 2007, p. 357). From the beginning of the seventeenth to the middle of the eighteenth century, the problematization of population that enabled happiness to be connected with the population was eventually made possible by 'a series of transformations thanks to which and through which this notion of population, which will be a kind of central element in all political life, political reflection, and political science from the eighteenth century, is elaborated' (Foucault 2007, p. 358).

The reflection of population on the basis of which the aim of reason of state in the seventeenth and eighteenth centuries became to ensure the happiness of its population was elaborated through a political technology/apparatus of police. Accord-

[26] This was also clearly expressed through the mercantilist politics in this period.

ing to Foucault (2007, p. 358) the apparatus of police 'was installed in order to make *raison d'État* function' (Foucault 2007, p. 358). Namely, in order to understand the role of the state in early modern society and its experience of happiness, we should not only focus on institutions and on the people who rule them, nor should we only analyze 'the theories or ideologies developed in order to justify or to legitimate the existence of the state' (Foucault 2002, p. 410). What is crucial to understand are the actual techniques, the practices, 'by which the individual could be integrated into the social entity' and which, thus, 'give a concrete form' to the political rationality of reason of state that constitutes the power axis of the early modern experience of happiness (Foucault 2002, p. 410).

Before we proceed, we have to note that since the nineteenth century, the concept of police has denoted a very specific institution that doesn't have much in common with the understanding of police in the early modern period when it had 'a very broad and, at the same time also a very precise meaning' (Foucault 2002, p. 410). Namely, in the seventeenth and eighteenth centuries, police corresponded to 'specific techniques by which a government in the framework of the state was able to govern people as individuals significantly useful for the world' (Foucault 2002, p. 410). In order to explain the police as a political technology of reason of state, Foucault (2002) depicts its manifestations in three major forms. The police started as a dream or utopia that eventually manifested in concrete political technologies and practices. Ultimately, it was even taught as an academic discipline.

In 1611, Luis Turquet de Mayerne published his utopian vision of an ideal universal technique of government that was highly representative of what this period deemed a well-governed state. According to Turquet, the task of the police 'was to foster civil respect and public morality' (Foucault 2002, p. 411), which should be carried out through four boards. The first board of police, Foucault explains (2002, p. 411), was 'to look after the positive, active, productive aspects of life'. Mainly, this board was 'concerned with education and with 'determining very precisely each individual's aptitudes and tastes,' which included a strict official categorization according to each person's aptitudes and occupation (Foucault 2002, p. 411). The second board, on the other hand, 'was to see to the negative aspects of life, that is, the poor, widows, orphans, the aged, who required help' (Foucault 2002, p. 411). In addition, it also had 'to take care of public health, diseases, epidemics, and accidents such as fire and floods, and it had to manage a kind of insurance for people to be protected against all such accidents'. The third board, Foucault further explains (2002, p. 411), was responsible for 'commodities and manufacturers' goods: it indicated what was to be produced and how. It also controlled markets and trading, which was a very traditional function of police'. And last but not least, the fourth board was concerned with 'territory, space, private property, legacies, donations, sales, and also to manorial rights, roads, rivers, public buildings, and so on' (Foucault 2002, p. 411).

According to Foucault (2002, p. 411), Turquet's text demonstrates that while 'the police appears as an administration heading the state together with the judiciary, the army, and the exchequer,' it in fact 'embraces all those other administrations'. The police, Turquet argues (in Foucault 2002, p. 411), 'branches out into all of the people's conditions, everything they do or undertake. Its fields comprise justice, finance, and the army' (Turquet 1611 in Foucault 2002, p. 412). In sum, Foucault explains (2002, p. 412), the police according to Turquet is concerned with 'live, active and productive man'; or, in Turquet's (in Foucault 2002, p. 412) own words: 'the police's true object is man'.

While Turquet's utopia did not explicitly posit happiness as the goal of police, the tasks of police that he proposed were concerned with the areas of human existence that were later clearly associated with happiness. Less than a century later, we can already find happiness clearly defined as the central object of police in Lamare's text on police (Traite de la police 1705). In addition, De Lamare's text is composed as a 'manual or systematic encyclopedia for the use of civil servants,' which testifies that the police were no longer only a political utopia, but a concrete political technology.

Covering roughly the same areas as Turquet's utopia, De Lamare understands police as basically seeing to everything. He organizes his encyclopedia of police under 11 chapters that correspond to 11 things that police have to ensure within the state: '(1) religion; (2) morals; (3) health; (4) supplies; (5) roads, highways, town buildings; (6) public safety; (7) the liberal arts (roughly speaking, arts and science); (8) trade; (9) factories; (10) manservants and laborers; (11) the poor' (De Lamare in Foucault 2002, p. 320). Similarly to Turquet, De Lamare also sees police as 'taking care of living' (Foucault 2002, p. 413).

Concerning the 11 areas of police intervention, Foucault explains (2002, p. 413), De Lamare makes the following remarks. The police are concerned with religion not from the standpoint of religious dogma or salvation in the afterlife, but more pragmatically from the viewpoint of 'the moral quality of life' (Foucault 2002, p. 321). Moreover, 'in seeing to health and supplies, it deals with the preservation of life; concerning trade, factories, workers, the poor, and public order—it deals with the conveniences of life' (Foucualt 2002, p. 321). And last but not least, the police also has to take care of the practices of pleasure such as theatre, literature and entertainment, which we have already described above. Taking care of living beings, the police, therefore, has to ensure both 'the indispensable, the useful, and the superfluous' (Foucault 2002, p. 413). In other words, the police has to see 'that people survive, that people live' and 'that people do even better than just survive or live' (Foucault 2002, p. 413). So what, then, is the sum total of the 11 objects of police, the cardinal goal of police? It is precisely happiness: 'The sole purpose of the police is to lead man to the utmost happiness to be enjoyed in this life,' De Lamare argues (in Foucault 2002, p. 321).

Within the political rationality of the reason of state, the connection between happiness and the state now acquires a new dimension. While 'from the beginnings of political philosophy in Western countries everybody knew and said that the happiness of people had to be the permanent goal of governments,' Foucault argues (2002, p. 413), happiness was conceived merely 'as the result or the effect of a really good government'. Due to the systematization of the French administrative practice prescribed by De Lamare, on the other hand, 'happiness is not only a simple effect. Happiness of individuals is a requirement for the survival and development of the state. It is a condition; it is an instrument and not simply a consequence'. Even more, people's happiness even 'becomes an element of state strength' (Foucault 2002, p. 414). Following from this, it is not surprising that the main thesis in De Lamare's book is 'that what is superfluous for individuals can be indispensable for the state, and vice versa' (Foucault 2002, p. 413).

The Biopolitics of Happiness

An even further development of the political technology of police can be observed in Germany, where police even became a discipline in the academic sense taught under the name of Polizeiwissenshaft. The most important written legacy of Polizeiwissenshaft is von Justi's Elements of Police, which is a kind of a manual for students of Polizeiwissenshaft. While, according to Foucault (2002, pp. 414–415), and similar to De Lamare, Von Justi also defines police 'as taking care of individuals in society,' he takes the political technology of police another step further by making 'an important distinction between what he calls police (die Polizei) and politics (die Politik)'. For Von Justi, politics is 'the negative task of the state' that involves 'the state's fighting against its internal and external enemies, using the law against the internal enemies and the army against the external ones' (Foucault 2002, p. 415). The police, on the other hand, has a positive task with the aim of 'permanently increasing production of something new, which is supposed to foster the citizens' life and the state's strength' (Foucault 2002, p. 415). As opposed to politics, the police 'govern not by law but by a specific, a permanent, and a positive intervention in the behavior of individuals[27]' (Foucault 2002, p. 415).

An illustrative example of typical police intervention and how it differs from justice governed by law can be found in Adam Smith's *Theory of Moral Sentiments*. 'If a person, Smith argues (2002, p. 120), 'should throw a large stone over a wall into a public street without giving warning to those who might be passing by, and without regarding where it was likely to fall, he would undoubtedly deserve some chastisement'. Considering that this person did not de facto break the law and 'had done no mischief' (Smith 2002, p. 120), of course he cannot be subject to legal punishment. This is where the police steps in. Namely, Smith (2002, p. 120) insists that 'a very accurate police' should 'punish so absurd an action' simply because 'the person who has been guilty of it shows an insolent contempt of the happiness and safety of others'.

---

[27] 'Even if the semantic distinction between Politik endorsing negative tasks and Polizei endorsing positive tasks,' explains Foucault (2002, p. 415), 'soon disappeared from political discourse and from the political vocabulary, the problem of a permanent intervention of the state in social processes,' is still 'characteristic of our modern politics and political problematics'. Namely the discussions from the end of the eighteenth century till now about issues such as liberalism and welfare state actually originate 'in this problem of the positive and negative tasks of the state, in the possibility that the state may have only negative tasks and not positive ones and may have no power of intervention in the behavior of people'.

Another crucial element of Von Justi's conception of police is his reflection of population 'that has been very influential with all the political and administrative personnel of the European countries at the end of the eighteenth century and the beginning of the nineteenth' (Foucault 2002, p. 415). Von Justi certainly did not invent the concept of population, but he was definitely the first who, under the name population, took 'what demographers were discovering at the same moment' and put it into the reflexive prism of political rationality of reason of state (Foucault 2002, p. 415). In this sense, Von Justi sees 'all the physical or economic elements of the state as constituting an environment on which population depends and which, conversely, depends on population' (Foucault 2002, p. 415). Insofar, according to Von Justi, 'the population and environment are in a perpetual living interrelation,' the state 'has to manage those living interrelations between those two types of living beings' (Foucault 2002, p. 415). Following from this, Foucault concludes (2002, p. 415), 'the true object of the police becomes, at the end of the eighteenth century, the population; or, in other words, the state has essentially to take care of men as a population. It wields its power over living beings, and its politics, therefore, has to be biopolitics' (Foucault 2002, p. 416). We could, therefore, say, that the power axis constituting the experience of happiness is essentially marked by biopolitics and that the modern experiences of happiness is, thus, always also a biopolitics of happiness.

While the cardinal aim of reason of state and police was initially the happiness of the state itself (Chemnitz), which then followed the happiness of man (De Lamare), towards the end of the eighteenth century, the cardinal aim of reason of state became the happiness of the population for Von Justi. This extension of the reflexive prism from the state to the population, however, is ultimately always folded back into the state, or better in favor of the state. Namely, the political rationality of reason of state begins taking the happiness first of man and then of the population into account only insofar as they are also starting to be perceived as a means that reinforce the state itself. Since in this sense 'the population is nothing more than what the state takes care of for its own sake,' the biopolitics of happiness can quickly also turn into what Foucault (2002, p. 416) calls 'thanatopolitics,' meaning that ultimately the state is even 'entitled to slaughter' its population, if it finds that necessary for its strength and preservation.

In this last section of the last chapter covering the power axis of the modern experience of happiness, we have tried to analyze how 'the modern Western state has integrated into a new political shape an old power technique that originated in pastoral institutions' (Foucault 2002, p. 332) and how this process was connected to the (birth of) experience of happiness.

Concomitant with the processes of secularization, the Church institution (through which pastoral power was exercised as part of the medieval experience of sin) was not eliminated, but replaced by state apparatuses and political technologies that began to constitute the power axis of the experience of happiness. As we have seen, in the seventeenth and eighteenth centuries, the power axis of the experience of happiness was characterized by political rationality of raison of state (and its political technology police) that were closely related to 'a new distribution, a new organization of this kind of individualizing power,' which was no longer exercised through the Church institution but through the modern state (Foucault 2002, p. 334). In line with the transformations introduced in the process of birth of happiness on the axes of truth and the relationship to the self, we can observe a clear change in the objective of this new form of pastoral power that now suddenly 'spread out into the whole social body' (Foucault 2002, p. 335):

> It was a question no longer of leading people to their salvation in the next world but, rather, ensuring it in this world. And in this context, the word "salvation" taken on different meanings: health, well-being (that is, sufficient wealth, standard of living), security, protection against accidents. A series of "worldly" aims took the place of the religious aims of the traditional pastorate, all the more easily because the latter, for various reasons, had followed in an accessory way a certain number of these aims; we only have to think of the role of medicine and its welfare function assured for a long time by the Catholic and Protestant churches (Foucault 2002, p. 334).

Similarly, as the pastoral power guided by the principle Omnes et Singulatim[28], on the substrate of which it sprouted, this new form of power is also both individualizing and totalizing.

Within the medieval experience of sin, the secular sovereign power only 'consisted in relations between juridical subjects insofar as they were engaged in juridical relations by birth, status, or personal engagement' (Foucault 2002, p. 413). With the new problematization of sovereignty manifested as the reason of state and police, the state begins adopting totalizing and individualizing functions exercised before exclusively by the pastoral institution. We first have the state government that in the seventeenth century 'begins to deal with individuals, not only according to their juridical status but as men, as working, trading, living beings' (Foucault 2002, p. 412). In the eighteenth century, we can then observe an evolution of political rationality, which starts governing men also as a population:

> From the idea that the state has its own nature and its own finality to the idea of man as living individual or man as a population in relation to an environment, we can see the increasing intervention of the state in the life of individuals, the increasing importance of life problems for political power, and the development of possible fields for social and human sciences insofar as they take into account those problems of individual behavior inside the population and the relations between a living population and its environment (Foucault 2002, p. 416).

On account of this, Foucault argues (2002, p. 417), the main characteristic of our modern political rationality 'is neither the constitution of the state,' nor 'the rise of bourgeois individualism'. Rather, the cardinal characteristic of modern political rationality 'is the fact that this integration of individuals in a community or in a totality results from a constant correlation between an increasing individualization and the reinforcement of this totality' (Foucault 2002, p. 417). Based on this political rationality is a form of power

[28] Above in the section about pastoral power we have argued that the principle Omnes et Singulatim implies that the pastor/shepherd does everything for the totality of his flock, but he does everything also for each sheep of the flock.

> that applies itself to immediate everyday life categorizes the individual, marks him by his own individuality. Attaches him to his own identity, imposes a law of truth on him that he must recognize and others have to recognize in him. It is a form of power that makes individuals subjects. There are two meanings of the word "subject": subject to someone else by control and dependence, and tied to his own identity by a conscience or self-knowledge. Both meanings suggest a form of power that subjugates and makes subject to (Foucault 2002, p. 331).

Insofar as the modern state represents 'a new form of pastoral power,' we should not simply consider it 'as an entity that was developed above individuals, ignoring what they are and even their very existence,' but, on the contrary, Foucault argues (2002, p. 334), 'as a very sophisticated structure in which individuals can be integrated, under one condition: that this individuality would be shaped in a new form, and submitted to a set of very specific patterns'. And these patterns are largely connected to the experience of happiness.

From this, it follows not only that the state as the new matrix of individualization is important for the understanding of experience of happiness, but also vice versa. Namely, happiness is also important for understanding of the (birth of) the modern state and its exercise of power, through which 'we have been led to recognize ourselves as a society, as a part of a social entity, as a part of a nation or of a state' (Foucault 2002, p. 404). A good example of this in the context of our discussion is the welfare state problem, which, according to Foucault (2002, p. 307), 'does not only bring the needs or the new governmental techniques of today's world to light,' but it must also 'be recognized for what it is: one of the extremely numerous reappearances of the tricky adjustment between political power wielded over legal subjects and pastoral power wielded over live individuals'.

And last but not least, it is important to note that the rise of this new political rationality and this new political technology should be also seen as closely connected to the emergence of social sciences (some of them were mentioned above). 'If man—if we, as living, speaking, working beings—became an object for several different sciences,' Foucault argues (2002, p. 417), 'the reason has to be sought not in an ideology, but in the existence of this political technology which we have formed in our own societies'. We believe that empirical quantitative happiness research that explicitly rests on the Enlightenment pursuit of (public) happiness should also be critically reflected in this light. After all, it takes the individualizing hermeneutical aspect of subjective well-being assessment and conjoins it with the collective aspect of national SWB comparisons in which the happiness of individuals and populations are recognized primarily in terms of the (national) state.

Chapter 7
The Evolution of Happiness: Development of Happiness from its Birth to its Contemporary Manifestations

The Christian experience of sin marked the refusal/sacrifice of the self that preceeded the experience of Happiness can be seen as a period in the history of Western thought characterized by what could be called a "negative constitution of the subject." Insofar as the birth of happiness was in large part constituted as a break away from the Christian experience of sin, the pursuit of happiness represents a refusal of this negative constitution of the subject. Instead, the experience of happiness from its initial eighteenth century outlook to its contemporary manifestations can be seen as closely connected to what Foucault (2000a) calls the positive constitution of the subject. Happiness understood in terms of a positive constitution of the subject, however, did not occur without retaining certain elements from the preceding experience of sin that are mostly related with the implicit sediments of the Christian hermeneutics of the self and the individualizing form of power closely related to it. Following from this, one of the great problems of Western culture largely connected to the birth of happiness 'has been to find the possibility of founding the hermeneutics of the self not, as it was the case in early Christianity, on the sacrifice of the self but, on the contrary, on a positive, on the theoretical and practical, emergence of the self' (Foucault 1999, p. 180). The main consequence of this development is that 'a hermeneutics of the self has been diffused across Western culture through numerous channels and integrated with various types of attitudes and experience, so that it is difficult to isolate and separate it from our own spontaneous experiences' (Foucault 2000a, p. 224).

Analyzing the axis of truth and the axis of power constituting the experience of happiness, we have seen that the "refusal of the negative Christian subject" was clearly the aim of the early modern (political) theory and practice, which aimed 'to constitute, positively, a new self' (Foucault 2000a, p. 249) (of happiness) 'in order to make of the individual a significant element of the state' (Foucault 2002, p. 409). In this sense the modern state represents a continuation of the individualizing and totalizing form of power connected to the hermeneutics of the self that was hitherto characteristic of the pastoral institution. This means that the 'power of a pastoral type, which over centuries—for more than a millennium—had been linked to a defined religious institution, suddenly spread out into the whole social body' and 'found support in a multitude of institutions' (Foucault 2002, p. 335). Such an

DOI 10.1007/978-3-319-04403-3_7,

individualizing tactic, then, 'characterized a series of powers: those of the family, medicine, psychiatry, education, and employers' (Foucault 2002, p. 335).

The new form of pastoral power exercised through the state as a 'modern matrix of individualization' (Foucault 2002, p. 334) was closely connected to the emergence of a positive self in 'the so-called human sciences' focused on the 'the development of knowledge of man around two roles: one, globalizing and quantitative, concerning the population; the other, analytical, concerning the individual' (Foucault 2002, p. 335). This resulted in reinserting the remains of the Christian hermeneutics (especially the techniques of verbalization) and the individualizing and totalizing form of power 'in a different context' (Foucault 2000a, p. 249) dominated on the one side by the judicial and political institutions and technologies and, on the other, by medical, psychiatric and educational institutions and practices.

The aim of constituting a positive self can also be observed on the axis of relationship to the self constituting the modern experience of happiness. In contrast to the negative Christian subject that had to neutralize desire for the sensual and "clean" the self through the hermeneutics of the self, the subject of happiness has to liberate and fulfill the desire in order to achieve happiness. The traces of Christian hermeneutics, however, remained. Namely, the desire is important in both modes of experience, which both put the individual in a position in which he never fulfills his moral obligations enough; he never surrenders enough. The Christian is never clean enough because—as we have seen earlier—there is always 'the possibility that Satan can get inside your soul and give you thoughts you cannot recognize as satanic' (Foucault 2000a, p. 270). Such circumstances require constant hermeneutical work. Similarly, the modern subject of happiness follows an external imperative to enjoy and to be happy, but never succeeds in being happy enough. The individual within the experience of happiness is—in contrast to his medieval ancestor—free to desire, but the model of the hermeneutics of the self and the internal tension remain. If the hermeneutic work imposed upon the Christian self aims to discover the root of desire in order to eradicate it, the hermeneutic work performed by the subject of happiness is used to discover the truth of desire in order to liberate it. This is necessary because akin to the Christian subject also in the subject of happiness, there is a constant internal uncertainty in which 'the very abstraction of happiness explains its seductive power and the anguish it produces' (Bruckner 2010, p. 4). 'Not only are we wary of prefabricated paradises,' Bruckner further explains (2010, p. 4), 'but we are never sure that we are truly happy. When we wonder whether we are happy, we are already no longer happy'.

While in the medieval period the wider effect of the Christian refusal and hermeneutics of the self was the glorification of suffering, the wider effect of the problematization of happiness and the remains of hermeneutics of the self in the modern experience of happiness ultimately resulted in what Bruckner (2010, p. 5) calls 'the duty to be happy'. According to Bruckner (2010, p. 5), the duty to be happy refers to the 'ideology' that 'urges us to evaluate everything in terms of pleasure and displeasure, a summons to a euphoria that makes those who do not respond to it ashamed or uneasy. A dual postulate: on the one hand, we have to make the most of our lives;

on the other, we have to be sorry and punish ourselves if we don't succeed in doing so'. In contemporary western societies it is possible to find numerous practices and techniques of happiness that range from consumer practices to therapy, training, self-help books and meditation that can all be potentially marked by compulsory happiness.

In order to demonstrate the relevance of the analysis of the origins of happiness for the understanding of its present day manifestations we shall now look more closely at the modern consumer practices that represent the dominant strategy of happiness in contemporary western culture.

Contemporary Compulsory Happiness and Consumer Culture

In the second half of the twentieth century, the rapid process of industrialization and commodification enabled an economic system and a consumer society with an almost unlimited supply of highly differentiated consumer goods with a plethora of cultural meanings attached to them, offering the average Western consumer a broad freedom of consumer choice (Featherstone 1991; Slater 1997). As such, contemporary consumer culture "is premised upon the expansion of capitalist commodity production which has given rise to a vast accumulation of material culture in the form of consumer goods and sites of purchase and consumption," and "has resulted in the growing salience of leisure and consumption activities in contemporary Western societies" (Featherstone 1991, p. 13).

Within the Foucauldian perspective, increased freedom (of choice) in the consumption realm means that the experience of the average consumer in contemporary Western societies has become determined less by the direct influence of external/objective conditions and more by the nature of one's relationship to oneself. For Foucault a complex historical experience is "constituted from and around certain forms of behavior: an experience that conjoins the field of knowledge," "a collection of rules (which differentiate the permissible from the forbidden, natural from monstrous, normal from pathological, what is decent and what is not, and so on)," "and a mode of relation between the individual and himself" (Foucault 2000, p. 200). O'Leary (2002, p. 36) explains that for Foucault "while these three axes constitute any matrix of experience, it is not the case that their relative importance is always the same." In the case of consumption in the pre-modern era, for example, commodities were largely distributed by "a collection of rules" (Foucault 2000, p. 200); that is, systems of coercion and concrete (physical) dividing practices. Most people consumed what was available or given to them according to their position in society and were thus more "passive subjects" (Foucault 2000, p. 291) of the consumption experience. Here it is important to note that many people in numerous developing countries and even certain marginalized, disadvantaged people in Western societies are still dependent on similar distribution strategies. We also do not argue that social status has completely lost its significance in contemporary society but, considering the vast supply of consumer goods, the predominating consumption patterns are directly enforced much less and are therefore more the result of a "mode of relation between the individual and himself" (Foucault 2000, p. 200). In this sense contemporary consumers are more "active subjects" who constitute themselves "in an active fashion through practices of the self" (Foucault 2000, p. 291). Nevertheless, these practices are "not something invented by the individual himself: They are models that he finds in his culture and are proposed, suggested, imposed upon him by his culture, his society, and his social group" (Foucault 2000, p. 291). Contemporary consumer practices are thus proposed as practices of the self ("*pratiques de soi*"), which in Western society largely constitute our present experience and which became an important strategy of the individual to construct his personal identity and make sense of the world in which he lives and acts. According to Foucault (2000, p. 87), self-forming activities are an important part of the relationship to oneself and can be defined as

> the procedures, which no doubt exist in every civilization, offered or prescribed to individuals in order to determine their identity, maintain it, or transform it in terms of a certain number of ends, through relations of self-mastery or self-knowledge.

These self-forming activities are important especially because they are "frequently linked to the techniques for the direction of individuals" (Foucault 2000 p. 277).

The Freedom to Consume and the Freedom to Desire

Freedom (in the consumption realm) therefore always comes at a price: "there is the way in which political argument bases itself increasingly upon the value of maximization of individual freedom and choice, and enjoins each person and family to take responsibility for the care of themselves" (Rose 1996, p. 295). As such, contemporary consumption practices are one of the "points of intersection between programmes for the government of others and the practical means accorded to human beings to understand and act upon themselves" (Rose 1996, p. 298). Such accounts of consumer practices are based on Foucault's concept of governmentality, with which he intended "to cover the whole range of practices that constitute, define, organize, and instrumentalize the strategies that individuals in their freedom can use in dealing with each other" (Foucault 2000 p. 300).

According to Binkley (2006), we have to be careful when applying the theory of governmentality to the realm of consumption, which has its own distinctive characteristics. For Binkley (2006, p. 343), theorists of governmentality like Rose, DuGay and Dean "who have assessed the various methods by which the personal freedoms imposed by neo-liberal social, economic and cultural configurations are instrumentalized, made the objects of direction and control" have "underemphasized the practices of the consumer, or reduced them to a dependent set of practices to that of professional, productive life." Binkley (2006) believes that such a theoretical undertaking is inappropriate because in the consumption realm different kinds of freedoms operate than in the production realm:

> Like the entrepreneur, the freedom of the consumer is the freedom to transform the self by stepping back in thought, but the medium of such thinking is not that of instrumental planning but of something quite different—it is one of fantasy, play, distraction and imaginary escape (Binkley 2006, p. 351).

In sum, Binkley argues that "the problem today is not merely the government of freedom, but the identification, separation and allocation of distinct modes of freedom to their respective realms" (Binkley 2006, p. 344). In the case of consumption this demands the unique adoption of the governmentality thesis for this particular realm:

> To better understand how consumption is governed, we must grasp the kinds of freedoms that operate within its domain—a freedom that is characterized less by instrumental behavior and more by expressive and ephemeral dispositions sustainable only in a bounded realm of liminality and play (Binkley 2006, p. 352).

At this point, we would like to extend Binkley's argument even further and propose that, just as there are distinctions in the modes of freedom between the production and the consumption realms, also within the consumption realm itself there are certain differences in the modes of freedom that demand their own specific theoretical accounts. Even though Binkley (2006, p. 352) considers the role of desire and imagination within the consumption realm, he remains focused on the aspect of freedom that we will name *the freedom to consume*. This aspect of freedom in the consumption realm is connected with the broad freedom of consumer choice in contemporary Western societies enabled by "a vast accumulation of material culture in the form of consumer goods and sites of purchase and consumption," (Featherstone 1991, p. 13) and intensified as the realm of consumption is becoming "radicalized in its magnitude and reach" (Binkley 2006, p. 345). The increasing "powers of seduction and aesthetization" in the consumption realm are induced by an "increasing elaboration of consumer media" and with the "easy availability of consumer credit" (Binkley 2006, p. 345). The perspective of the *freedom to consume* subsumes predominately external conditions that are supposed to determine individuals consuming experience and the risks within it:

> The increasingly persuasive powers of consumption, from physical environments to media, have generated a culture that undermines rational pattern of thinking, exposing individuals to currents of desire that often motivate purchasing decisions that are inconsistent with their larger needs, budgets and other responsibilities (Binkley 2006, p. 355).

From this point of view, consumers are confronted with powerful external seductions and thus need to be equipped with a new "technique of governmentality," a "unique modality of selfcontrol and discipline" in the form of various "therapeutic treatments" aimed at preventing them from "losing themselves entirely" in the "phantasmagorical transformations of the carnivalesque" (Binkley 2006, p. 355). Consumers have to learn how "to withstand seductions without giving in entirely to them" (Binkley 2006, p. 355). As such, "the binding of the liminal constitutes an object of governmentality itself" (Binkley 2006, p. 355). According to Binkley what is of great importance here are the boundaries between the various realms of freedom: "The responsibilized subject is one capable of disentangling the modes of autonomous choice that operate in these realms, and consigning each to their respective logics of government" (Binkley 2006, p. 344). Individuals in contemporary consumer societies therefore have to "learn the tricks of maintaining boundaries between production and consumption as a personal responsibility" (Binkley 2006, p. 359). In addition to Binkley's perspective, which is clearly an important contribution to the theory of consumption as well as to the field of governmentality studies, we believe that there is another more internal and subjective aspect of freedom operating in the realm of consumption: *the freedom to desire*. In order to fully understand how the conditions for the contemporary consumption experience are constituted, it is not enough to only consider the external factors like the extensive supply of consumer goods or the easy availability of consumer credit, but we also have to remember Rose (1996, p. 295) and take into account that "subjectivity has its own history." As a consequence, we will conduct a genealogical analysis of freedom of desire, which is at the same time a genealogy of an important part of contemporary (consumer) subjectivity. While the analysis of the freedom to consume is best undertaken with the help of Foucault's concept of governmentality (which is well stated by Binkley (2006)), we believe that Foucault's concept of ethics provides us with a better theoretical perspective for the analysis of the freedom to desire. Obviously desire is also present within the freedom to consume but, from that perspective, it is not the desire itself that is problematic as are the material consequences of the consumer's decisions caused by it. While within the freedom to consume individuals are incited to govern themselves in order to avoid the material and pathological consequences of their "currents of desire" (Binkley 2006, p. 355, 356), within the freedom to desire they are jeopardized by desire itself. The freedom of desire is not only problematic because it motivates possible irresponsible and irrational consumer behavior, but also because it can—through the modern hermeneutics of the self—cause permanent internal tension within contemporary modes of consumer subjectivity. As such, while the possible dangerous consequences of the freedom to consume can be harmful mostly in extreme cases (like compulsive shopping), the dangers of the freedom to desire connected with the modern hermeneutics of the self are acute in a broader sense, since "a hermeneutics of the self has been diffused across Western culture through numerous channels and integrated with various types of attitudes and experience, so that it is difficult to isolate and separate it from our spontaneous experience" (Foucault 2000, p. 224). Foucault's genealogical analysis along four aspects of ethics (relationship to oneself) reveals that Christianity, with its emphasis on the practices of the renunciation of the self, in comparison with antiquity, has brought certain internal tensions to Western forms of subjectivity. As a consequence, we see the main danger of freedom to desire in its potential to present a continuity of certain elements of Christian forms of subjectivity that could in a similar way also create internal tensions for modern individuals seeking happiness through consumption.

Can Consumption Really Bring Happiness?

As we have argued above in the contemporary Western forms of subjectivity there remain traces of Christian self-renunciation and the techniques of hermeneutics of the self. In order to understand how in spite of the fact that the other aspects of the relationship to oneself have undergone significant transformations the techniques of self-deciphering have only been modified slightly, we will now examine the contemporary (consumer) self.

Ethical substance for modern individuals is, according to Foucault (2000, p. 263), constituted by the realm of feeling itself. In the case of the modern consumer self, it is especially the feelings of happiness and pleasure that are emphasized. The telos is no longer beyond our world in heaven like for the Christians but in this very world of the here and now. The feeling of happiness, which in the modern consumer society is closely related with desire, is emphasized even so much that the French philosopher Pascal Bruckner (2000, p. 16) speaks of compulsory happiness:

> I understand compulsory happiness as an ideology of the second half of the twentieth century, which judges everything only according to pleasure or displeasure it brings to our experience, as a command that we have to be euphoric. Everyone who doesn't subject to it has to be ashamed and forced into a feeling of discomfort.

This moral responsibility of the absolute happiness and self-fulfillment connected with pleasure and joy that preferably should last for the whole life is a consumer's mode of subjectivation. The desire is important in both subjectivation processes (Christian and consumer) which both put the individual in a position in which he never fulfils his moral obligations enough, he never surrenders enough. The Christian is never clean enough because as we saw earlier that there is always "the possibility that Satan can get inside your soul and give you thoughts you cannot recognize as satanic" (Foucault 2000 p. 270). Such circumstances require constant hermeneutical work. Similarly, the modern consumer follows an external imperative to enjoy and to be happy, but never succeeds in being happy enough. The desire is now emancipated: "I could say that the modern formula is desire, which is theoretically underlined and practically accepted, since you have to liberate your own desire" (Foucault 2000, p. 269). The individual is now free to desire but the practice of the hermeneutics of the self and the internal tension remain. If the hermeneutic work imposed upon the Christian self aims to discover the root of desire in order to eradicate it, the hermeneutic work performed by the consumer self is used to discover the truth of desire in order to liberate it. This is necessary because, similarly as in the Christian self, in the consumer self there is a constant internal uncertainty. In the consumer case this is about whether real happiness can be achieved by consuming. When we try to liberate our desire by consuming there is a permanent tension connected with the following questions and doubts: When we buy a certain consumer product, does it bring enough happiness to us? Could we be even happier? Are we truly happy? Do we have to be happier? Can we really find self-fulfillment in consuming? Is there something with the product that might jeopardize our feeling of happiness? Should we have bought another product? And so on. As a consequence, in practice every actual acquisition of a consumer commodity finally leads to disappointment, which in turn starts to feed new desire. Out of the immanent implicit concern that real products would again disappoint him, the desire itself and not the actual objects become the predominant source of pleasure for the modern consumer. According to Colin Campbell's *Romantic Ethic and the Spirit of Modern consumerism* (1996), modern consumer hedonism is not so much about materialism and the appropriation of goods but about seeking pleasure in the imagination. For Campbell (1996, p. 203), modern consumer ethics is marked:

> by a preoccupation with pleasure, envisaged as a potential quality of all experience. In order to extract this from life, however, the individual has to substitute illusory for real stimuli, and by creating and manipulating illusions and hence the emotive dimension of consciousness, construct his own pleasurable environment. This modern, autonomous, and illusory form of hedonism commonly manifests itself as day-dreaming and fantasizing.

And the more the consumer relies on imagination and desire as the main source of pleasure, the more he gets disappointed with the actual acquisition of real goods, and so the circle continues. Since material objects never provide absolute fulfillment, the modern consumer instead starts to take pleasure in practices of imagination, which are closely connected with the modern hermeneutics of the self and present a continuity of Christian technology of the self. Imagining, desiring and fantasizing about consumer commodities are always closely related with the hermeneutics of the truth about our desire, needs and self-fulfillment.

As we have seen, the problem of desire is central for the Christian self as well as for the consumer self. If the Christian form of subjectivity urged the individual to suppress his desire in order to achieve the telos (absolute purity), then the situation with the consumer mode is exactly the opposite but finally leads to very similar hermeneutical technologies of the self. The telos for the consumer self requires the constant fulfillment and actualization of desire, which results in an essential and for the consumer constitutive paradox: the more he strives to fulfill his desire through the consumption of material objects, the further away he moves from materialism itself. If Christians suppressed their desire in order to distance themselves from worldly material goods, the modern consumer achieves the same outcome through the inflation of desire. But this does not mean that the modern consumer does not spend. Indeed this distance from the material is merely an internal process, which results in another paradox. The internal distance from the material world can produce even greater material consequences in the economic realm since the products used as stimulators of the imagination and impulsive shopping are needed in even greater numbers than objects with their use value only[1].

[1] Critical debates around contemporary consumer culture and its relation to happiness can also be found in the field of happiness studies and (positive) psychology. In his book *The High Price of Materialism* Kasser (2002) uses empirical data to show that excesive materialism and consumerism can have negative effects on well-being. *Psychology and consumer culture: The struggle for a good life in a materialistic world, book* edited by Kasser and Kanner (2012) devoted to the relationship between materialism and well-being from a psychological perspective is also worth mentioning here. In addition to psychology some researchers are also dealing with this topic from the perspective of economics (see for example Helliwell 2003).

Chapter 8
Conclusion: Modernization as the Collective Pursuit of Happiness

Trying to illuminate the birth of happiness in Western culture occurring in the seventeenth and the eighteenth centuries, the genealogical analysis began way back in the period of the early institutionalization of Christianity. The main reason for such a wide chronological focus was that in order to understand the birth of happiness as one of the decisive breaks in the history of Western thought, it is first necessary to understand the experience that preceded it. Above, we have seen not only in many respects that the experience of happiness was constituted in relation to the preceding experience of sin, but also that there are certain important continuities between the two modes of experience. In short, the modern experience of happiness in Western culture would not have had emerged as it did and would certainly not have the same specifics if it hadn't been for the Christian experience of sin from which it tried to break away.

In line with the new interdisciplinary approach to the study of happiness that was developed in Chap. 3, the genealogical analysis was conducted along the three axes that, according to Foucault, constitute the historical a priori of experience in a particular area of human existence: the axis of truth, the axis of relationship to the self and the axis of power.

Analysis of the axis of truth first explored how Christianity established the truth about salvation as the cardinal ideal of human existence and why such an ideal wasn't achievable in the present life. According to the official Christian doctrine established by the Council of Carthage in 418 (presided by St. Augustine), the main inhibition not allowing humans to experience true bliss (or Christian perfection) already in this life was Adam's original sin. The Church professed that Original sin stained all humanity, rendering humans incapable of controlling their will, which resulted in mortality and in inevitable breaching of God's commandments. Through the problematization of salvation, the ideal of human existence was connected to heaven in the afterlife where the chosen ones would be immersed in eternal bliss (lat. beatitudo).

While throughout the Middle Ages there indeed were certain disagreements in the Christian realm about what heaven as the ideal of human existence will be like, this dispute 'never occupied center stage in Christian polemics' (Walls 2002, p. 34). What, however, has been 'seriously contested,' Walls explains (2002, p. 34), 'is how

L. Zevnik, *Critical Perspectives in Happiness Research*,
DOI 10.1007/978-3-319-04403-3_8,

to get to heaven'. Following from this, the analysis of the axis of truth constituting what we have called the Christian experience of sin was mainly focused on the tension between the tragic consequences of original sin and the capacity of free will, which is essentially concerned with the degree to which humans can contribute to the ideal of human existence by their own efforts. At one extreme, there was the Augustinian radical refusal of free will according to which salvation can only be bestowed by the mercy of God, and on the other there was the Pelagian total acceptance of free will perceived as the gift from God, which held that it is possible to achieve Christian perfection entirely by human efforts.

While in the first two centuries after the Pelagian polemic the Augustinian version (at least officially) prevailed, we have seen that from its very beginning it was never completely accepted in the Christian realm. In fact, (especially) after the Carolingian renaissance in the ninth century, there was a clear trend of gradual reinforcement of the idea of free will that was later further elaborated by Aquinas and the Renaissance movement. In light of this trend (which never actually went all the way to the Pelagian extreme, though), Christianity from the ninth to the sixteenth centuries officially and practically endorsed the idea of free will according to which humans can/should to a certain degree contribute to their salvation by their own efforts. This resulted in the ideas and practices of treasury of merit, the hierarchy of the sacred and the glorification of suffering, which significantly marked Christian life within the experience of sin and which were eventually challenged by the Reformation movement in the sixteenth century.

The focus on the tension between the tragic consequences of original sin and the capacity of free will has proved relevant because the theme directly or indirectly fueled the majority of central theological polemics in the Christian realm, culminating in the Reformation movement. With the help of the idea of original sin, it was also possible to explain why the ideal of Christian existence was not achievable already in this life. At the same time, this also helped to reveal the main aspect that later had to be refused if the ideal of human existence was to be positioned in the present life and if it was to become entirely achievable by human efforts.

In addition, such focus has illuminated the gradual trend of reinforcement of free will that represented an important process later contributing to the birth of happiness in two ways. In a more direct way, it first—at least partly—contributed to the start of the problematization of (good) feeling in the present life within the Renaissance movement and later in the seventeenth century constituted one of the aspects (besides the affirmation of everyday life) in the Deist convergence, which explicitly refused original sin and proclaimed the ideal of human existence as being entirely achievable by human efforts already in the present life. More indirectly, the current of reinforcement of free will contributed to the birth of happiness by producing theological views on justification, concrete practices and social patterns that represented the main points of controversy, kindling the Reformation movement, which—amongst other things—caused the affirmation of everyday life that eventually constituted the second main aspect of the Deist convergence.

And last but not least, analyzing the question of how to reach heaven rather than what heaven will be like has enabled us to explore more thoroughly how the ideal of existence envisioned in the afterlife has practically influenced Christian life in this world. Namely, the analysis of the other two axes constituting the Christian experience of sin has shown that the Christian problematization of salvation was fundamentally marked by what Foucault calls Christian hermeneutics of the self, which implies the refusal and the sacrifice of the self. This "negative constitution of the subject" produced two major effects for the Christian experience of sin. At the level of the relationship to the self and practices of the self, the Christian subject constituted through practices of self-deciphering (such as confession), publication of the self and self-mortification had to neutralize the desire for sensual pleasures that in a more general sense resulted in the privileged status of earthly suffering in the Christian tradition. On the axis of power, the Christian hermeneutics of the self and self-deciphering connected to the vision of salvation was employed to institutionalize a new form/technology of power that was totalizing and individualizing. This 'pastoral power' governed 'men in their daily life on the grounds of leading them to eternal life in the other world' and operated through 'a mode of individualization by subjection (assujettissement)' (Foucault 2007, p. 199, p. 239).

We have concluded the analysis of the Christian problematization of salvation and the concomitant experience of sin by arguing that they cannot be simply equated with the (modern) problematization and experience of happiness, which only emerged in the seventeenth and eighteenth centuries, when the ideal of human existence increasingly started to be pursued in the present life.

The first steps towards the birth of happiness can be traced back to the Renaissance and the Reformation movement, which were still, however, mainly characterized by the problematization of salvation and the Christian experience of sin. In addition to the existent and still prevalent problematization of salvation, the Renaissance movement (starting in the fifteenth and sixteenth centuries) and the Reformation movement (starting in the sixteenth century) introduced what we have called the problematization of (good) feeling and the affirmation of everyday life, which later resulted in the problematization and experience of happiness. The problematization of (good) feeling on earth and the affirmation of everyday life for some time, therefore, coexisted with the preceding and still dominant problematization of salvation, until in the seventeenth century the former started to slowly but surely dominate the latter. We have argued that it was precisely this transformation (in which good feeling on earth in connection with the affirmation of everyday life started becoming the primary ideal of human existence) that represented the first major development, which marked the birth of the modern experience of happiness. The second such major development was that the ideal of human existence not only became possible already in this world, but also that it became perceived as entirely achievable with human efforts. It is crucial to note that these two major developments not only mark the birth of happiness, but also represent the two major characteristics or parameters of modern experience of happiness that at the same time also fundamentally distinguish it from the preceding experience of sin.

The processes of the birth of happiness produced two main modes of the modern experience of happiness. Still retaining certain elements of (Christian) divinity, we have called the first manifestation of happiness the religious experience of happiness. The cardinal development that enabled the problematization of (good) feeling in connection with the affirmation of everyday life to become dominant was the refusal of original sin, which hitherto represented the main inhibition not allowing human to achieve the ideal of human existence already in the present life. On the axis of truth, the idea of original sin was questioned by natural theology and Deist philosophy, which represent a convergence of the rationalist current of affirmation of free will, the Protestant affirmation of everyday life and the problematization of (good) feeling/pleasure. The refusal of (original) sin was closely connected to two decisive developments, which marked the birth of happiness and can be at the same time considered as the main parameters of the modern experience of happiness: (a) via the reinforcement of the problematization of (good) feeling the ideal of human existence started to be positioned primarily in this life and (b) the ideal of human existence started to be perceived as entirely achievable with human efforts.

Completely neutralizing the tragic consequences of original sin, the rationalized Christianity promoted the idea of divine providential order created by God for the harmonious well-being and happiness of its inhabitants both in this world and in the world to come (provided that they lived in accordance with God's laws and commandments). The transposition of the universalizing Christian logic of sin to the universalizing idea of (the possibility) of happiness inherent in the idea of divine providential order virtually enabled for the first time in the history of Western thought the preparation of the ground for the understanding of the ideal of human existence on earth (i.e. happiness) also in collective terms, which later culminated in the Enlightenment idea of public happiness. The Deist convergence, also closely accompanied by wider social developments, slowly but surely transformed the common religious outlook to increasingly understand God primarily as a foundation for happiness on earth.

In addition to the religious experience of happiness less than a century later, a secular experience of happiness also emerged as part of the continuation of the process of the birth of happiness in Western culture. Being largely connected to secularization catalyzed by the Enlightenment movement, it represents a logical evolution of the initial religious experience of happiness except that it completely eliminates the explicit residue of (Christian) divinity hitherto still serving as the foundation for happiness. Following from this, the divine providential order intrinsically created for the harmonious well-being of its inhabitants is replaced by the neutral natural causalities that have to be rationally deciphered and used accordingly for the maximization of pleasure and the minimization of pain. Using the idea of harmony of interest now based on the glorification and idealization of rationality rather than on the preceding idea of divine providential order, the principle of utility is then also widened to guide not only the individual, but also the collective pursuit of happiness. Believing that both individual and public happiness cannot rely on a pre-existing providential order and even further radicalizing the idea that the ideal of human existence (i.e. happiness) is achievable entirely by human efforts, the mainstream Enlightenment current intrinsically connected the utilitarian ideal of human happiness with scientific, technological, individual, social, political and economic progress[1].

In regard to the understanding of the inherent human drive for pleasure and its role in the relation between individual and collective/public happiness, the secular experience of happiness conjoins two conflicting aspects. On the one hand, we have the dominant rationalistic-utilitarian aspect that promotes public happiness, which through the idea of harmony of interest encompasses individual and communal happiness based on the principle of utility and, on the other hand, we have the amoral mode of egoistic hedonism that advocates unrestrained expression of the individual instinctive drive for pleasure. We have argued that the tension between these two aspects significantly influences the constitution of experience of happiness on all three axes of experience.

In sum, the historical a priori of a possible experience of happiness constituted on the axes of truth, power and relationship to the self is therefore manifested in the form of two main modes of experience of happiness: the religious experience of happiness and the secular experience of happiness. This a priori of experience, then, sets the shared basic parameters of experience of happiness within which the majority of strategies of happiness and individual experiences of happiness emerged and still continue to emerge in Western culture.

[1] Even though the book focuses on the period ranging from the fourth to the eighteenth centuries, in light of future research it is worth noting that in the nineteenth century it is possible to observe certain (mostly intellectual) movements that questioned particular aspects of the Enlightenment project of progress towards (public) happiness. In direct contrast to the medieval material scarcity, low overall quality of life and Christian refusal of sensual pleasures, initially the dominant strategies of happiness were predominantly tied to emphasizing material welfare, economic progress and physical sensual gratification. Marxism was the first influential intellectual movement that criticized the exploitation of large segments of the population in the context of the industrial revolution and the unequal distribution of the fruits of material progress for which the Enlightenment movement believed that is supposed to unquestionably contribute to public happiness. On the other hand, romanticism at roughly the same time questioned the widespread Enlightenment assumption that material welfare, rationalism and physical gratification alone can bring happiness (this is at least partly related to the fact that the romantics were mostly wealthy aristocrats well acquainted with the abundance of sensual pleasures); hence the romantic emphasis on intimacy, emotions and "weltschmerz". Another important intellectual movement in the nineteenth century that can be considered as a sort of questioning of the Enlightenment vision of happiness was psychoanalysis. While for the romantics physical gratification alone is not enough to bring true happiness, for Freud physical gratification cannot be simply equated with happiness because it is ultimately impossible. We have argued that for the mainstream Enlightenment vision of the pursuit of (public) happiness, an individual on his own or society (if he is not capable of doing so) ought to rationally restrain the inherent individual drive for pleasure (what Freud (1961) calls 'the pleasure principle'). On the contrary for Freud in *Civilization and Its Discontents* (1961), it is precisely this "civilized restraining" of desire that is the main source of unhappiness (in Freudian terms, pleasure principle vs. reality principle). It is true that Freud (1961) sees the origins of this tension as emerging much earlier than in the eighteenth century. Nevertheless, we believe that the early experience of happiness and its vision of public happiness can be seen as a development in Western thought that can help us understand—to a certain extant at least—the context in which Freud started to problematize this tension.

To conclude, the genealogy of the birth of happiness provides relevant new contributions for the study of happiness. First and foremost, it helps us to understand the process of the cultural and historical constitution of the experience of happiness in Western culture and its basic parameters. In turn, this also supports the argument from the first part of the book according to which happiness should not be understood in a universal sense, but as a culturally and historically specific/singular notion and experience in Western culture that is tightly connected with the relations of power in society. Insofar as the birth of happiness constituted a basic structure for all the later forms of experience of happiness in Western culture, we think that the next important contribution of our analysis is that it represents a valuable point of departure for any further inquiries into manifestations of happiness (including its research) in our culture. And last but not least, we believe that the examination of the birth of happiness is also valuable in a wider sense by indicating that happiness has represented one of the central themes guiding the modernization processes that fundamentally determine what we experience today. Following from this, the understanding of (the birth of) happiness is essential in terms of representing a broader context in which, or as a part of which, important aspects of individual and social life such as consumer culture, the modern state, economic system, science and technology, influential intellectual movements, etc. have emerged in the West. The Enlightenment idea of progress and the modernization processes connected to it can, therefore, be effectively seen in the context of the pursuit of happiness and, as such, as integral parts of the experience of happiness in the West. Ever since the birth of the secular experience of happiness in the eighteenth century, progress in Western culture has essentially been tantamount to progress towards happiness.

Bibliography

Positive Psychology Center faq. 2010. Accessed http://www.ppc.sas.upenn.edu/faqs.htm.

Ahmed, Sara. 2007/2008. The happiness turn. *New Formations* 63:1–14.

Ahmed, Sara. 2010. *The Promise of Happiness*. Durham: Duke University Press.

Allestree, Richard. 1677. *The art of contentment*. Oxford. http://books.google.com/books?id=4SI3AAAAMAAJ&dq=allestree+richard+the+art+of+contentment&source=gbs_navlinks_s. Accessed 2011.

Aquinas, Thomas. 2006. *Summa Theologica: Project Guttenberg*.

Augustine, of Hippo. 1994. *The confessions of saint augustine*. Hyde Park: New City Press.

Augustine, of Hippo. 2006. *The confessions of saint augustine*. Fairfield: 1stworldlibrary.com.

Augustine, of Hippo. 2007. *Beata Vita, edited by S. M. Cahn and C. Vitrano*. Oxford: Oxford University Press.

Augustine, of Hippo. 2009. City of God: Digireads.com Publishing.

Bagchi, David. 2000. Luther's catholic opponents. In *The reformation world*, ed. A. Pettegree. London: Routledge.

Barker, Chris. 2000. *Cultural studies: Theory and practice*. London: Sage.

Barker, Chris. 2002. *Making sense of cultural studies: Central problems and critical debates*. London: Sage.

Barker, Chris. 2004. *The SAGE dictionary of cultural studies*. London: Sage.

Barret, Stanley. 1996. *Anthropology: A student's guide to theory and method*. Toronto: University of Toronto Press.

Baumeister, Roy F. 1991. *Meanings of life*. New York: Guilford.

Beccaria, Cesare. 1986. *On crimes and punishment*. Indianapolis: Hackett.

Beeke, Joel R. 2004. Calvin on piety. In *The Cambridge companion to John Calvin*, ed. D. K. McKirn. Cambridge: Cambridge University Press.

Bentham, Jeremy. 1817. *A table of the springs of action: Hunter*. http://books.google.com/books?id=XmVBAAAAcAAJ&dq=a+table+of+the+springs+of+action&source=gbs_navlinks_s. Accessed 2011.

Bentham, Jeremy. 1969. A fragment on government. In *A Bentham Reader*, ed. P. M. Mack. New York: Pagasus.

Bentham, Jeremy. 1983. *Deontology together with a table of the springs of action and the article on utilitarianism*. Oxford: Clarendon Press.

Bentham, Jeremy. 2000. *An introduction to the principles of morals and legislation*. Kitchener: Batoche Books.

Beutel, Albrecht. 2003. *Luther's life. In the Cambridge companion to Martin Luther*, ed. D. K. McKirn. Cambridge: Cambridge University Press.

Binkley, Sam. 2007. Governmentality and lifestyle studies. *Sociology Compass* 1:111–126.

Binkley, Sam, and Jorge Capetillo-Ponce, eds. 2009. *Foucault for the 21st century: Governmentality, biopolitics and discipline in the new millennium*. Newcastle upon Tyne: Cambridge Scholars Publishing.

L. Zevnik, *Critical Perspectives in Happiness Research*,
DOI 10.1007/978-3-319-04403-3,

Bruckner, Pascal. 2001. *L'euphorie perpétuelle: Essai sur le devoir de bonheur*. Paris: B. Grasset.

Bruckner, Pascal. 2010. *Perpetual euphoria: On the duty to be happy*. Princeton: Princeton University Press.

Bruni, Luigino, and Pier Luigi Porta, eds. 2007. *Handbook on the economics of happiness*. Cheltenham: Edward Elgar Publishing Limited.

Burchell, Graham, Colin Gordon, and Peter Miller, eds. 1991. *The foucault effect: Studies in governmentality*. Chicago: Chicago University Press.

Burckhardt, Jacob. 1945. *The civilization of the renaissance in Italy*. Oxford: Phaidon.

Burton, Robert. 1621. *The anatomy of Melancholy: Project guttemberg*. http://www.gutenberg.org/ebooks/10800. Accessed 2011.

Cacioppo, J. T, L. C. Hawkley, A. Kalil, M. E Hughes, L. Waite, and Thisted. R. A. 2008. Happiness and the invisible threads of social connection: The Chicago health, aging, and social relations study. In *The science of subjective well-being*, ed. M. Eid and R. J. Larsen. New York: Guilford Press.

Cahn, Steven M, and Christine Vitrano. 2008. *Happiness: Classic and contemporary readings in philosophy*. New York: Oxford University Press.

Calamy, Edmund. 1662. *The happinesse of those who sleep in Jesus, or, the benefit that comes to the dead bodies of the saints even while they are in the grave, sleeping in Jesus*. Westminster: N. Webb.

Calvin, John. 1975. *John Calvin: Selection from his writings*. Oxford: Oxford University Press/Scholars Press.

Calvin, John. 2002. *The Institutes of the christian religion*. Grand Rapids: Christian Classics Ethereal Library.

Cantril, H. 1965. *The pattern of human concern*. New Brunswick: Rutgers University Press.

Christopher, John C. 1999. Situating psychological well-being: Exploring the cultural roots of its theory and research. *Journal of Counseling & Developement* 77:141–152.

Classen, Albrecht, and Marilyn Sandidge, eds. 2008. *Sexuality in the middle ages and early modern times: New approaches to a fundamental cultural-hisotrical and literary-anthropological theme*. Berlin: Walter de Gruyter.

Clifford, James. 1986. On ethnographic allegory. In *Writing culture:The poetics and politics of ethnography*, ed. J. Clifford and G. E. Marcus. Berkley: University of California Press.

Clifford, James, and George E Marcus, eds. 1986. *Writing culture: The poetics and politics of ethnography*. Berkley: University of California Press.

Cottingham, John. 1998. *Philosophy and the good life. Reason and the passions in Greek, Cartesian and psychoanalytic ethics*. Cambridge: Cambridge University Press.

Couzens Hoy, David, ed. 1986. *Foucault: a critical reader*. Oxford: Blackwell.

Cowburn, John. 2008. *Free will, predestination and determinism*. Milwaukee: Marquete University Press.

Davidson, Arnold. 1986. Archeology, genealogy, ethics. In *Foucault, a Critical Reader*, ed. D. Couzens Hoy. Oxford: Blackwell.

Davidson, Richard J., Urry L. Heather, Jack B. Nitschke, Isa Dolski, Daren C. Jackson, Kim M. Dalton, Corrina J. Mueller, Melissa A. Rosenkranz, Carol D. Ryff, and Singer H. Burton. 2004. Making a life worth living: Neural correlates of well-being. *American Psychological Society* 15(6): 367–372.

Davies, Brian. 1992. *The thought of Thomas Aquinas*. Oxford: Clarendon Press.

De Mirandola, Pico. 1496. *De Hominis Dignitate: Progetto Pico*. Bologna: Universita degli Studi di Bologna & Brown University. http://www.brown.edu/Departments/Italian_Studies/pico/index.html. Accessed 2011.

Derham, William. 1711. *Physico-theology: or, A demonstration of the being and attributes of God*. London. http://books.google.com/books?id=jp8 PAAAAIAAJ&printsec=frontcover&dq=William+Derham&hl=en&ei=_ORYTYD8EtS64ganhs2lBw&sa=X&oi=book_result&ct=result&resnum=1&ved=0CCYQ6AEwAA#v=onepage&q&f=false. Accessed 2011.

Diener, Ed. 1984. Subjective well-being. *Psychological Bulletin* 95:542–575.

Diener, Ed. 2007. Culture and subjective well-being. In *Handbook of cultural psychology*, ed. S. Kitayama and D. Cohen. New York, London: The Guilford Press.

Diener, Ed, and Robert Biswas-Diener. 2008. *Happiness: Unlocking the mysteries of psychological wealth*. Oxford: Blackwell Publishing.
Diener, Ed, and Shigehiro Oishi. 2000. Money and happiness: Income and subjective well-being across nations. In *Culture and subjective well-being*, ed. E. Diener and E. M. Suh. Boston: The MIT Press.
Diener, Ed, and Eunkook M Suh, eds. 2000. *Culture and subjective well-being*. Boston: The MIT Press.
Diener, Ed, M Suh Eunkook, and Shigehiro Oishi and. 1997. Recent findings on subjective well-being. *Indian Journal of Clinical Psychology* 24(1): 25–41.
Dilenberger, John. 1975. An Introduction to John Calvin. In *John Calvin: Selection from his writings*, ed. J. Dilenberger Scholars Press.
Dohmen, Joep. 2003. Philosophers in the "art-of-living". *Journal of Happiness Studies* 4:351–371.
Eid, Michael, and Randy J. Larsen, eds. 2008. *The science of subjective well-being*. New York: The Guilford Press.
Erasmus, Desiderius. 1969. *De Libero Arbitri. In Luther and Erasmus: Free Will and Salvation*, ed. G. Rupp, A. N. Marlow, P. S. Watson and B. Drewery. Philadelphia: Westminster Press.
Erasmus, Desiderius. 2008. *The praise of folly*. Rockville: Arc Manor.
Esterlin, Richard A. 1974. Does economic growth improve the human lot? Some empirical evidence. In *Nations and households in economic growth: essays in honor of Moses Abramovitz*. Waltham: Academic Press.
Foucault, Michel. 1978. *The history of sexuality: Volume I: An introduction*. New York: Pantheon Books.
Foucault, Michel. 1979. *Discipline and punish: The birth of the prison*. New York: Vintage.
Foucault, Michel. 1980. *Power/knowledge: Selected interviews and other writings*. New York: Pantheon.
Foucault, Michel. 1983. *The culture of the self: Recorded lecture*. Berkley.
Foucault, Michel. 1988. *Politics philosophy culture: Interviews and other writings 1977–1984*. New York: Routledge.
Foucault, Michel. 1990. *The use of pleasure: Volume 2 of the history of sexuality*. New York: Vintage Books.
Foucault, Michel. 1994. *The order of things: An archeology of human sciences*. New York: Vintage Books.
Foucault, Michel. 1999. *Religion and culture: Michel Foucault*. New York: Routledge.
Foucault, Michel. 2000a. *Essential works of Foucault Vol. 1: Ethics*. London: Penguin.
Foucault, Michel. 2000b. *Essential works of Foucault Vol. 2: Aesthetics*. London: Penguin.
Foucault, Michel. 2001. *Fearless speech*. Los Angeles: Semiotext(e).
Foucault, Michel. 2002. *Essential works of Foucault Vol. 3: Power*. London: Penguin.
Foucault, Michel. 2004. *The archeology of knowledge*. London. Routledge.
Foucault, Michel. 2005. *The hermeneutics of the subject*. New York: Picador.
Foucault, Michel. 2006. *History of madness*. Oxon: Routledge.
Foucault, Michel. 2007. *Security, territory, population: Lectures at the college de France, 1977–78*. Hants: Palgrave Macmillan.
Foucault, Michel. 2008. *The birth of biopolitics: Lectures at the college de France*. London: Palgrave Macmillan.
Freud, Sigmund. 1961. *Civilization and its discontents*. New York: Norton & Company Inc.
Fromm, Erich. 1981. Primary and secondary process in waking and in altered states of consciousness. *Academic Psychology Bulletin* 3:29–45.
Fromm, Erich. 2007. *To have or to be?* New York: Continuum.
Geertz, Clifford. 1973. *The interpretation of cultures*. New York: Basic Books.
Gowland, Angus. 2006. *The worlds of renaissance melancholy: Robert Burton in context*. Cambridge: Cambridge University Press.
Kaspar von Greyerz. 2008. *Religion and culture in early modern Europe*. Oxford: Oxford University Press.
Gros, Frederic. 2005. *Course context. In the hermeneutics of the subject, ed.* A. Davidson. New York: Picador.

Hadot, Pierre. 1995. *Philosophy as a way of life*. Oxford: Blackwell Publising.

Haidt, Jonathan. 2006. *The happiness hypothesis: Putting ancient wisdom and philosophy to the test of modern science*. Random House: Arrow Books.

Hall, Stuart, ed. 1999. *Representation: Cultural representations and signifying practice*. London: Sage.

Hall, Stuart, ed. 1999. The work of representation. In *1999. Representation: cultural representations and signifying practice*, ed. Stuart Hall. London: Sage.

Helliwell, John. 2006. Well-being, social capital and public policy: what's new? *The Economic Journal* 116:510 (Conference Papers pp. 34–45).

Harper, Douglas. 2011. *Online etymology dictionary* 2011. Accessed http://www.etymonline.com/.

Holbach, P H. 1761. *Christianity unveiled: Being an examination of the principles and effects of the christian religion.*

Holbach, P H. 1966. *Le Systeme de la Nature*. Hildesheim: Georg Olms.

Holbach, P H. 1995. *Common sense, or natural ideas opposed to supernatural.* In *The Portable Enlightenment, ed.* I. Kramnick. New York: Penguin.

Huizinga, Johan. 1987. *The waning of the middle ages*. London: Penguin Books.

Israel, Jonathan I. 2001. *Radical enlightenment: philosophy ans the making of modernity 1650–1750*. Oxford: Oxford University Press.

Jacobs, Alan. 2008. *Original Sin, A Cultural History: Harper Collins e-books.*

Johnson, Samuel. 1805. *Rasselas*. London: William Miller. http://books.google.com/books?id=r8tBAAAAYAAJ&printsec=frontcover&dq=rasselas&hl=en&ei=hPhYTal_xIHkBoudgKcH&sa=X&oi=book_result&ct=result&resnum=2&ved=0CCsQ6AEwAQ#v=onepage&q&f=false. Accessed 2011.

Kahneman, Daniel, Ed Deiner, and Norbert Schwartz, eds. 1999. *The foundations of hedonic psychology*. New York: Russel Sage Found.

Kant, Imanuel. 2011. *An answer to the question: What is enlightenment?* 17842011]. Accessed http://www.english.upenn.edu/~mgamer/Etexts/kant.html.

Kant, Imanuel. 2009. *An answer to the question: What is enlightenment?* London: Penguin.

Kashdan, T.B., R. Biswas-Diener, and L.A. King. 2008. Reconsidering happiness: The costs of distinguishing between hedonics and eudaimonia. *Journal of Positive Psychology* 3:219–233.

Kasser, Tim. 2002 *The high price of materialism*. Cambridge: MIT Press.

Kasser, Tim (Ed), Allen D. Kanner, ed. 2004. *Psychology and consumer culture: The struggle for a good life in a materialistic world.* Washington, DC: American Psychological Association.

Kekes, John. 1995. *Moral wisdom and good lives*. Ithaca: Cornell University Press.

Kekes, John. 2002. *The art of life*. Ithaca: Cornell University Press.

Kent, Bonnie. 2006. *Augustine's ethics.* In *The Cambridge companion to Augustine*, ed. E. Stump and N. Kretzmann. Cambridge: Cambridge University Press.

Kent, W. 1910. *Indulgences.* In *The Catholic Encyclopedia.* New York: Robert Appleton Company.

Kerrigan, Michael. 2001. *The instruments of torture*. New York: The Lyons Press.

Kitayama, Shinobu, and Dov Cohen, eds. 2007. *Handbook of cultural psychology*. New York: The Guilford Press.

Kitayama, Shinobu, and Hazel R Markus. 2000. *The pursuit of happiness and the realization of sympathy: Cultural patterns of self, social relations, and well-being.* In *Culture and subjective well-being*, ed. E. Diener and E. M. Suh. Boston: The MIT Press.

Kraye, Jill. 2007. *Moral philosophy.* In *The Cambridge history of renaissance philosophy*, ed. *Q. Skinner and E. Kessler*. Cambridge: Cambridge University Press.

Kreeft, Peter. 1992. *Back to virtue*. San Francisco: Ignatius Press.

Kretzmann, Norman, Anthony Kenny, and Pinbork Jan, eds. 2008. *The Cambridge history of later medieval philosophy*. Cambridge: Cambridge University Press.

Kringelbach, M. L., and K. C. Berridge (2010). The neuroscience of happiness and pleasure. *Social Research: An International Quarterly* 77(2):659–678.

La Mettrie, J. 1994. *Man a machine and man a plant*. Indianapolis: Hackett.

La, Roche, and V. Sophie. 1933. *Sophie in London 1786, being the diary of Sophie v. La Roche*. London: Jonthan Cape.

Layard, Richard. 2006. *Happiness: Lessons from a new science*. London: Penguin.
Le Goff, Jacques. 1990. *The birth of purgatory*. Hants: Scolar Press.
LeVine, Robert A. 2007. *Anthropological foundations of cultural psychology*. In *Handbook of cultural psychology*, ed. S. Kitayama and D. Cohen. New York: The Guilford Press.
Lindberg, Carter. 2003. Luther's struggle with social-ethical issues. In *The Cambridge companion to Martin Luther*, ed. D. K. McKirn. Cambridge: Cambridge University Press.
Locke, John. 1979. *An essay concerning human understanding*. Oxford: Oxford University Press.
Locke, John. 1993. A letter concerning toleration. In *Political writtings of John Locke,* ed. Wootton. New York: Mentor Books.
Locke, John. 1996. *Some thoughts concerning education*. Indianapolis: Hackett.
Locke, John. 2008. Of civil government: The second treatise. Rockville: Wildside Press.
Lohr, C. H. 2008. The medieval interpretation of aristotle. In *The Cambridge history of later medieval philosophy,* ed. N. Kretzmann, A. Kenny and P. Jan. Cambridge: Cambridge university Press.
Lowe, E J. 2002. *Routledge philosophy guidebook to locke in human understanding*. New York: Routledge.
Lu, Luo, and Robin Gilmour. 2004. Culture and conceptions of happiness: Individual oriented and social oriented SWB. *Journal of Happiness Studies* 5:269–291.
Luther, Martin. *Vorrede auff die Epistel s. Paul: an die Romer*, 2011 1545. Accessed www.iclnet.org/pub/resources/text/wittenberg/german.bible/rom-eng.txt.
Luther, Martin. 1969. *De Servo Arbitrio. In Luther and Erasmus: Free Will and Salvation*, ed. G. Rupp, A. N. Marlow, P. S. Watson and B. Drewery. Philadelphia: Westminster Press.
Lyotard, Jean-Francois. 1984. *The postmodern condition: A report on knowledge*. Manchester: Manchester University Press.
Machiavelli, Niccolo. 2005. *The prince*. New York: Oxford University Press.
Marcus, George E, and Michael M J Fischer. 1986. *Anthrpology as cultural critique: an experimental moment in the human sciences*. Chicago: The University of Chicago Press.
Marshall, Peter. 2009. *The reformation*. Oxford: Oxford University Press.
Martin, Lynn A. 2001. *Alcohol, sex, and gender in late medieval and early modern europe. hampshire*. New York: Palgrave.
Marx, Karl. 1982. *Capital: A critique of political economy: Vol. I.* Middlesex: Penguin.
Mathews, Gordon, and Carolina Izquierdo, eds. 2009. *The pursuits of happiness well-being in anthropological perspective*. Oxford: Berghahn Books.
McDougall, Sara. 2008. The prosecution of sex in late medieval troyes. In *Sexuality in the middle ages and early modern times: New approaches to a fundamental cultural-hisotrical and literary-anthropological theme*, ed. A. Classen and M. Sandidge. Berlin: Walter de Gruyter.
McGrath, Alister E. 2003. *A brief history of heaven*. Malden: Blackwell Publising.
McGrath, Alister E. 2004 *Intelectual origins of the european reformation*. Malden: Blackwell Publising.
McKendrick, Neil, John Brewer, and J H Plumb. 1985. *The birth of a consumer society: The commercialization of 18th-Century*. England: Indiana University Press.
McKirn, Donald K, ed. 2003. *The Cambridge companion to Martin Luther*. Cambridge: Cambridge University Press.
McKirn, Donald K, ed. 2004. *The Cambridge companion to John Calvin*. Cambridge: Cambridge University Press.
McMahon, Darrin M. 2006. *Happiness: A history*. New York: Grove Press.
Mourant, A John, and J. Collinge William. 1992. *Saint Augustine: Four anti-pelagianwritings*. Washington D.C: The Catholic University of America Press.
Nehamas, Alexander. 1998. *The art of living: socratic reflections from Plato to Foucault*. Berkley: University of California Press.
Nettle, Daniel. 2006. *Happiness: The science behind your smile*. Oxford: Oxford University Press.
Nettle, Daniel. 2008. Introduction. In *happiness: classic and contemporary readings in philosophy*, ed. S. M. Cahn and C. Vitrano. New York: Oxford University Press.

Newman, Lex, ed. 2007. *The Cambridge companion to Locke's "essay concerning humanunderstanding"*. Cambridge: Cambridge University Press.

Nietzsche, Friedrich. 1873. *Schopenhauer as Educator*.

Nietzsche, Friedrich. 1968. *The will to power: Attempt at a revaluation of all values*. New York: Vintage.

Nietzsche, Friedrich. 1989. *On the genealogy of morals and Ecce Homo*. New York: Vintage.

Nietzsche, Friedrich. 1997. *Untimely meditations Cambridge texts in the history of philosophy*. Cambridge: Cambridge University Press.

Nietzsche, Friedrich. 2002. *Beyond good and evil: Prelude to a philosophy of the future*. Cambridge: Cambridge University Press.

Nussbaum, Martha. 1994. *Therapy of desire. Theory and practics in hellenistic ethics*. Princeton: Princeton University Press.

O'Leary, Timothy. 2002. *Foucault: The art of ethics*. New York: Continuum.

O'Leary, Timothy. 2008. Foucault, experience, literature. *Foucault Studies* (5):5–25.

O'Leary, Timothy. 2010. *Rethinking experience with Foucault*. In *Foucault and philosophy*, ed. T. O'Leary and C. Falzon. Oxford: Wiley-Blackwell.

O'Leary, Timothy, and Christopher Falzon, eds. 2010. *Foucault and philosophy*. Oxford: Wiley-Blackwell.

Oishi, Shigehiro. 2000. *Goals as cornerstones of subjective well-being: Linking individuals and cultures*. In *Culture and subjective well-being*, ed. *E. Diener and E. M. Suh*. Boston: The MIT Press.

Oishi, S., J. Graham, S. Kesebir, and I. C. Galinha. 2013. Concepts of happiness across time and cultures. *Personality & Social Psychology Bulletin* 39 (5): 559–577.

Ostroot, Nathalie, Doh Shin, and Wayne Snyder. 1982. Quality of life perceptions in two cultures. *Social Indicators Research* 11:113–138.

Ouweneel, Piet, and Ruut Veenhoven. 1991. *Cross-national differences in happiness: Cultural bias or societal quality*. In *Contemporary issues in cross-cultural psychology*, ed. *N. Bleichrodt and P. J. Drenth*. Amsterdam: Swets & Zeitlinger.

Pavot, William, and Ed Diener. 1993. Review of the satisfaction with life scale. *Psychological Assessment* 5:164–172.

Pettegree, Andrew, ed. 2000. *The reformation world*. London & New York: Routledge.

Pflug, Jan. 2009. Folk theories of happiness: A cross-cultural comparison of conceptions of happiness in Germany and South Africa. *Social Indicators Research* 92:551–563.

Plato. 2003. *The republic, Cambridge texts in the history of political thought*. Cambridge: Cambridge University Press.

Porter, Roy. 1996. Enlightenment and pleasure. In *Pleasure in the eighteenth century*, ed. R. Porter and M. Mulvey Roberts. Houndmills: Macmillan Press.

Porter, Roy. 1996. *Material pleasures in the consumer society*. In *Pleasure in the eighteenth century*, ed. R. Porter and M. Mulvey Roberts. Houndmills: Macmillan Press.

Porter, Roy, and Marie Mulvey Roberts, eds. 1996. *Pleasure in the Eighteenth Century*. Houndmills: Macmillan Press.

Rabinow, Paul. 1986. *Representations are social facts: Modernity and post-modernity in anthropology*. In *Writing culture:The poetics and politics of ethnography*, ed. J. Clifford and G. E. Marcus. Berkley: University of California Press.

Ray, John. 1691. *the wisdom of god manifested in the works of creation*. http://www.jri.org.uk/ray/wisdom/. Accessed 2011.

Rickless, Samuel C. 2007. Locke's Polemic against Nativism. In *The Cambridge Companion to Locke's "essay concerning human Understanding"*, ed. L. Newman. Cambridge: Cambridge University Press.

Roche, Daniel. 2000. *A history of everyday things: The birth of consumption in France 1600–1800*. Cambridge: Cambridge University Press.

Rorty, Richard. 1979. *Philosophy and the mirror of nature*. Princeton: Princeton University Press.

Rothschild, Emma. 2001. *Economic sentiments: Adam Smith, condorcet and the enlightenment*. Cambridge: Harvard University Press.

Rupp, Gordon, A N Marlow, Philip S Watson, and B Drewery, eds. 1969. *Luther and Erasmus: free will and salvation*. Philadelphia: Westminster Press.
Ruut, Veenhoven. 1997. Advances in understanding happiness. *Revue Québécoise de Psychologie* 18:29–74.
Ryan, Richard M., and Edward L. Deci. 2000. Self-determination theory and the facilitation of intrinsic moti- vation, social development, and well-being. *The American psychologist* 55:68–78.
Ryan, Richard M. 2001. On happiness and human potentials: A review of research on hedonic and eudaimonic well-Being. *Annual Review of Psycholo*gy (52):141–166.
Ryff, CD, and CLM Keyes. 1995. The structure of psychological well-being revisited. *Journal of Personality and Social Psychology* 69:719–727.
Ryff, Carol D. 1995. Psychological well-being in adult life. *Currunt Directions in Psychological Sciences* 4:99–104.
Schaff, Philip. 1899. *The seven ecumenical councils: Christian Classics Ethereal Library*. http://www.ccel.org/ccel/schaff/npnf214.html. Accessed 2010.
Schofield, Philip. 2006. *Utility and democracy: The political thoughtof Jeremy Bentham*. Oxford: Oxford University Press.
Selingman, Martin E. P. 2003. *Authentic happiness: using the new positive psychology to realize your potential for lasting fulfillment*. London: Nicholas Brealey Publishing.
Skinner, Quentin, and Eckhard Kessler, eds. 2007. *The Cambridge history of renaissance philosophy*. Cambridge: Cambridge University Press.
Smith, Adam. 2002. *The theory of moral sentiments*. Cambridge: Cambridge University Press.
Smith, Adam. 2007. *An inquiry into the nature and causes of the wealth of nations*. Hampshire: Harriman House.
Stachniewski, John. 1991. *The persecutory imagination: English puritanism and the literature of religious dispair*. Oxford: Clarendon Press.
Stump, Eleonore, and Norman Kretzmann, eds. 2006. *The Cambridge companion to Augustine*. Cambridge: Cambridge University Press.
Taylor, Charles. 2001. Sources of the Self: The making of the modern identity. Cambridge: Harvard University Press.
Taylor, Chloe. 2009. *The culture of confession from Augustine to Foucault: A genealogy of the 'confessing animal'*. New York, London: Routledge.
Thomas, Keith. 2009. *The ends of life: roads to fulfulment in early modern England*. Oxford: Oxford University Press.
Tiberius, Valerie. 2004. Cultural differences and philosophical accounts of well-being. *Journal of Happiness Studies* 5:293–314.
Toland, John. 1702. *Christianity not mysterious*. London. http://books.google.com/books?id=m5YCAAAAQAAJ&printsec=frontcover&dq=Christianity+Not+Mysterious&hl=en&ei=f2JVTZbYDsHM4gaOl4TXBg&sa=X&oi=book_result&ct=result&resnum=2&ved=0CDIQ6AEwAQ#v=onepage&q&f=false. Accessed 2011.
Triandis, Harry C. 2000. *Cultural syndromes in subjective well-being*. In *Culture and subjective well-being*, ed. E. Diener and E. M. Suh. Boston: The MIT Press.
Trinkaus, Charles E. 1965. *Adversity's noblemen: The italian humanists on happiness*. New York: Octagon Books.
Tyler, Stephen A. 1986. *Post-modern ethnography: From document of the occult to occult document*. In *Writing culture: The poetics and politics of ethnography*, ed. *J. Clifford and G. E. Marcus*. Berkley: University of California Press.
Uchida, Yukiko, Vinai Norasakkunkit, and Shinobu Kitayama. 2004. Cultural constructions of happiness: Theory and empirical evidence. *Journal of Happiness Studies* 5:233–239.
Valla, Lorenzo. 1977. *De Voluptate*. New York: Abaris.
Veenhoven, Ruut. 2006. Sociology's blind eye for happiness. In *16th World Congress of Sociology 2006*. Durban.
Voltaire. 1764. Bien, Souverain bien. In *Dictionnaire de Philosophie*.
Voltaire. 2006. *Candide and other stories*. Oxford: Oxford University Press.
Walls, Jerry L. 2002. *Heaven: The logic of eternal joy*. Oxford: Oxford University Press.

Waterman, AS. 1993. Two conceptions of happiness: contrasts of personal expressiveness (eudaimonia) and hedonic enjoyment. *Journal of Personality and Social Psychology* 64:678–691.

Wetzel, James. 2006. Predestination, pelagianism, and foreknowledge. In *The Cambridge companion to augustine,* ed. E. Stump and N. Kretzmann. Cambridge: Cambridge University Press.

Wierzbicka, A. 2004. Happiness in cross-linguistic & cross-cultural perspective. *Daedalus* 133 (2): 34–43.

White, Nicholas. 2006. *A brief history of happiness*. Oxford: Blackwell Publishing.

Wieland, Georg. 2008. Happiness: the perfection of man. In *The Cambridge history of later medieval philosophy,* ed. N. Kretzmann, A. Kenny and P. Jan. Cambridge: Cambridge University Press.

Williams, Raymond. 1983. *Keywords: A vocabulary of culture and soceity*. New York: Oxford University Press.

Wilson, Catherine. 2007. The moral epistemology of Locke's essay. In *The Cambridge Companion to Locke's "Essay concerning human Understanding"*, ed. L. Newman. Cambridge: Cambridge University Press.

Wriedt, Markus. 2003. Luther's theology. In *The Cambridge companion to Martin Luther,* ed. D. K. McKirn. Cambridge: Cambridge University Press.

Zevnik, Luka. 2009. The consumer hermeneutics of the self and modern compulsory happiness. In *Foucault for the 21st Century: Governmentality, Biopolitics and Discipline in the New Millennium*, ed. S. Binkley and J. Capetillo-Ponce. Newcastle upon Tyne: Cambridge Scholars Publising.

Zevnik, Luka. 2010. Towards a new perspective in cultural studies: Emotional and spiritual problems and happiness in contemporary Western societies. *International Journal of Cultural Studies* 13(4).

Index

L. Zevnik, *Critical Perspectives in Happiness Research,*
DOI 10.1007/978-3-319-04403-3, © Springer International Publishing Switzerland 2014